Parenting ADHD

Proven Therapeutic Strategies to Empower Your Child With ADHD, Working Together to Strengthen Their Academic and Social Skills

Gerarld Paul Clifford

© Copyright 2020 by Gerarld Paul Clifford. All rights reserved.

The work contained herein has been produced with the intent to provide relevant knowledge and information on the topic described in the title for entertainment purposes only. While the author has gone to every extent to furnish up to date and true information, no claims can be made as to its accuracy or validity as the author has made no claims to be an expert on this topic. Notwithstanding, the reader is asked to do their own research and consult any subject matter experts they deem necessary to ensure the quality and accuracy of the material presented herein.

This statement is legally binding as deemed by the Committee of Publishers Association and the American Bar Association for the territory of the United States. Other jurisdictions may apply their own legal statutes. Any reproduction, transmission or copying of this material contained in this work without any written consent of the copyright holder shall be deemed as a copyright violation as per the current legislation in force on the date of publishing and subsequent time thereafter. All additional works derived from this material may be claimed by the holder of this copyright.

The data, depictions, events, descriptions and all other information forthwith are considered to be true, fair and accurate unless the work is expressly described as a work of fiction. Regardless of the nature of this work, the Publisher is exempt from any responsibility of actions taken by the reader in conjunction with this work. The Publisher acknowledges that the reader acts of their own accord and releases the author and Publisher of any responsibility for the observance of tips, advice, counsel, strategies and techniques that may be offered in this volume.

Table of Contents

Introduction..8
Statistics and Facts..11
Chapter 1: Basics of ADHD................... 13
ADHD and Its Causes................................... 13
ADHD and Heredity 15
Anatomy of The Brain.............................. 17
Other Related Factors 18
Symptoms of ADHD......................................18
Hyperactivity and Impulsivity................ 19
Inattention.. 20
ADHD and Its Types 21
Primarily Inattentive ADHD................... 21
Primarily Hyper-Active Impulsive Disorder... 21
Combination ADHD................................22
Diagnosis of ADHD 22
ADHD and Its Treatments 25
Medication..26
Therapy 28
Chapter 2: Common Myths About ADHD 30
ADHD Cannot Be Regarded As a Real Disorder... 30
ADHD Is Often Over-Diagnosed..................32
ADHD Can Only Be Found In Children......33
ADHD Is the Result of Bad Parenting 35
One of the Surest Symptoms of ADHD Is Hyperactivity 35
People Suffering From ADHD Cannot Focus At All..36

Stimulants Might Result in Addiction and Drug Abuse 37
Medication Can Completely Treat ADHD .. 37
ADHD Develops When Children Are Lazy .38

Chapter 3: Opting for Self-Care 41
Concentrating on the Related Advantages .42
Teaching Your Child to Follow Through on Their Commitments 45
Working on Skills of Organization 45
Implementation of Pets to Teach Responsibility 47
Practicing Color Coding 48
Helping Your Child to Prepare Routines 49
What Is the Importance of Routine? 49
How Can a Routine Be Developed? 50
Assisting Them to Deal With Difficulties While Dressing Up 54

Chapter 4: ADHD Reinforcements 57
Accommodation 58
Attention 64
Avoidance 67
Antagonism 70
Acquisition 71

Chapter 5: Getting Knowledge About Self-Control 73
Helping Them to Connect Behavior With Consequence 73
Channelizing Your Child's Energy in Productive Things 76
Teaching Your Child to Follow Directions .. 77
Work on Enhancing Your Child's Listening Skills 81
Instilling Problem Solving Skills 83

Chapter 6: Practical Tips for Dealing With Problems in School 86

Enhancing Social Skills 86
  Teaching the Required Skills and
  Practicing *87*
  Enhancing Social Awareness *88*
  Working on Development of Friendship 89
  Working With School for Making the
  Status of Peer Better *90*
  How Can Teachers Help in Enhancing
  Social Competencies? *91*
Rules and Expectations Needs to Be Realistic
....93
Managing Distractibility 96
Management of Impulsivity 97
Reduction of Interruptions 99
Management of Hyperactivity 100
Making the Task of Learning Fun.............102

Chapter 7: Managing ADHD Behavior Outside the Boundary of School........ 105
Traveling By Car... 105
How to Deal With Your Child's Bad Behavior in Public Settings?...................................... 110
  Why Does ADHD Children Act Out? *110*
  Reasons Why ADHD Children Throw
  Tantrums... *111*
  Strategies to Deal With Tantrums *112*
Helping Your ADHD Child in Group Situations..115

Chapter 8: Using Medication for Treating ADHD...................................119
Stimulant Medicines 121
Non-Stimulant Medicines......................... 122

Chapter 9: Suggestions and Tips for Parenting ADHD Child 125
Making It Interesting 125

Teaching Time Management 126
Reminding Yourself That It Is Not Only Your Child Who Misbehaves.............................. 127
Approaching a Specialist for Getting Support 128
Being Calm 129
Conclusion 130

Introduction

I would like to congratulate you on purchasing *Parenting ADHD*, and thanks a lot for doing so.

Mental health is of prime importance, no matter what your age is. In this section, you will be getting knowledge about the concept of ADHD that you require to know about before you move ahead to the more complex segments of this book. Attention Deficit Hyperactivity Disorder is the full form of ADHD. Well, as you can understand by the term ADHD, people with ADHD tend to showcase impulsive behaviors. They also tend to be hyperactive abnormally. It is considered to be a primary mental health disorder where people suffering from the same find it tough to sit still in one place for a long time and also cannot concentrate on any work or task that they are doing. Proper knowledge and awareness regarding this problem can help people get to know about ADHD in a better way and also opt for the help that they require. It has been found that ADHD is most commonly found in children. With the help of proper medication, it is possible to manage ADHD. However, the problem cannot be cured.

As already said, ADHD can be widely found in children; it is often regarded as a neurodevelopmental disorder. The most common age to get diagnosed with this disorder is seven years. Additionally, an interesting fact about ADHD is that it can be most commonly found in boys in comparison to girls. In fact, the symptoms can be found in adults as well. During the initial days, ADHD was not called by this name. It used a tougher term – hyperkinetic impulse disorder. Right after that, it got classified by the American Psychiatric Association or APA under the umbrella of mental disorder by the end of the 1960s. Well, ADHD came across various milestones. Here is a timeline description for you so that you can get a better hold of the history of the same.

- In the year 1902, ADHD came into being for the very first time. During that time, ADHD was only referred to as a minor defect in children that was regarded to be abnormal and affected their moral control. The description of ADHD was provided by a pediatrician, Sir George Still.
- The next milestone in the history of ADHD was in the year 1936 when FDA approved Benzedrine. However, right in the next year, the medicine started showing some kind of side effects. When children were provided with this medicine, their overall behavior and performance in school reached new heights of improvement. But all these

findings were not given any attention at that time.
- In the very first DSM edition, ADHD was not even referred to in the mental disorder category. It was in the year 1952 when the first edition came out. Right after that, in the year 1968, the second edition of DSM got published. In this edition, hyperkinetic impulse disorder made its name in the list.
- By the end of 1955, people started having some kind of idea about the nature of ADHD. FDA approved Ritalin, the drug, in that year. Ritalin is used even today.
- In the year 1980, DSM got its third edition published. In that edition, the term attention deficit disorder or ADD was put into use for the very first time instead of hyperkinetic deficit disorder. Because of this list, two ADD subtypes were formed. They were – ADD with hyperactivity and ADD without hyperactivity.
- In the year 1987, a revised DSM edition was published. The term ADHD was put into use for the first time finally.
- In the year 2000, the fourth edition of DSM was released, which included three ADHD subtypes-
  1. Combined types of ADHD
  2. Predominantly inattentive ADHD

3. Predominantly hyperactive-impulse ADHD

Statistics and Facts

Right before we delve deeper into ADHD, let's have a look at some quick facts regarding ADHD that you should definitely know about-

- In the lifetime of human beings, nearly 4.3% of women get diagnosed with ADHD. However, the percentage is quite high in the case of men at 13.2%.
- In comparison to women, men have higher chances of developing the symptoms of ADHD. The chances of men developing ADHD is three times more than that of women.
- There is no fixed rule that ADHD can affect only during childhood. American people deal with problems of ADHD even during their adulthood. According to statistics, about 5% of adults are above the age mark of 18 years that suffer from ADHD.
- If you calculate it in average, most people get diagnosed with the symptoms of ADHD by the age of 7 years.
- The symptoms of ADHD first start to appear between the ages of 3 and 6.

There are some other important facts that you need to know.

- Every race in the world gets affected by ADHD. But during the time span of 2001 – 2010, some sudden surge was noticed in non-Hispanic origin in black girls. The increase of ADHD affecting people of that race had an increase of almost 90%.
- 9.5% of Black children, 5.5% of Latino children, and 9.7% of White children get affected by ADHD.
- Although the numbers might differ from one state to the other, approximately 6.2% of American children are living under medication of ADHD and are also undergoing treatment. However, about 24% of American children are not getting treatment, medication, or counseling of any kind for ADHD.
- Approximately 6.5 million American children have been diagnosed with symptoms of ADHD. The age range is between 4 and 17.

There are several books on this subject available in the market. Thanks again for selecting this one! Every effort was made to make sure it is filled with as much useful information as possible; please enjoy!

Chapter 1: Basics of ADHD

Do you have the feeling that your child is having ADHD, however, you cannot be sure of it? If yes, then you are in the proper place, as we will discuss the basics of ADHD in this chapter. You will also gain knowledge whether your child is suffering from the same or not. In case your child is having trouble controlling their impulses and is hyperactive all the time, then the chances are high that he/she is suffering from the symptoms of ADHD. However, there are some other symptoms as well that you will have to look out for. As already discussed in the introduction, ADHD is much common in boys in comparison to girls. If not taken care of and when it makes its way into adulthood, ADHD can easily push someone towards addiction, relationship problems, or even breed in very low self-esteem. Keep reading to learn in detail about the various faces of ADHD.

ADHD and Its Causes

Right before we start discussing the various types of symptoms of ADHD, it is essential to first learn about what causes the same. There is a wide range of factors that tend to dedicate to this problem. However, the majority of researchers suggest that this neurodevelopmental disorder is mostly a genetic disorder right at the core. We all have a part of the brain which serves the function of 'executive functioning.' When any child is suffering from ADHD, that specific part of the brain gets affected. It can be considered as the primary reason why all those children suffering from this disorder find it difficult to showcase the correct emotions, plan their future, evaluate all their behaviors, control hyperactive impulses, or solve problems. The various types of challenges that can be found in any type of family because of the problems arising from ADHD might often make you forget the facts. If the problem gets escalated, it might seriously affect the behavior of the child in their classroom along with their personal relationships too.

There are parents who tend to believe that the problems came up as there was some kind of problem in their parenting style. Also, there are people who tend to assume that this neurodevelopmental disorder might be the result of some kind of traumatic event that took place in the life of their child during the early years or any kind of stressful or negative event that they were a part of. In fact, teachers who are not much aware of the problem or who do not tend to understand the intensity of the problem might also label the student as lazy or disobedient. However, if you really want to put forward your helping hand to someone who is suffering from this problem, be it an adult or a child, you will have to start by gaining knowledge about the root of this disorder. It is true that genetic factor is a definite reason behind the onset of ADHD. But you will have to remember that the blame does not have to be necessarily put on the parents of the child suffering from ADHD as they cannot do anything regarding the same.

ADHD and Heredity

There are a group of parents who all have one common question in their minds- "Is ADHD hereditary or not?" Well, the answer to this very question is yes. ADHD is hereditary. It can be regarded as a typical disease or disorder that tends to run in families. For the last thirty years, a huge number of research has been conducted to find out more details about ADHD. If you want to keep a count there, till now, there have been more than two thousand studies that have been conducted. Researchers are keeping up with their studies to get to know the real character of ADHD. Psychiatrists, psychologists, and geneticists all have worked on finding out more about this disorder. The majority of the time, you will see that a child who is suffering from ADHD will surely have someone in his/her family, be it their own parents or some other blood relative, who also had ADHD.

Various types of genes have been identified till now. All of them are most likely to be linked with the disorder. However, to properly specify the accurate genetic markers, more studies are still being conducted on this very subject. If you want to consider what has been found till now, it has been found that it is not only one gene that is solely responsible for this. However, you should also know that no genetic tests have been conducted till now in relation to ADHD. Also, there are a lot of misunderstandings that if a child is at risk of developing symptoms of ADHD genetically, it does not indicate that he/she will definitely have the same. There are various cases where kids did not develop ADHD while having the disorder in their family. Even there are cases where children developed ADHD when there is no existence of the same in their family. As there exists some kind of hereditary link of ADHD, some parents often feel guilty as they believe it was them who brought forward the disorder in their child.

It has also been found that when there is a child with ADHD in a family, about 25% of the family relatives have also shown the various symptoms of the disorder. The rate is quite higher in comparison to a family that did not have anyone suffering from ADHD. Also, if a parent has twins who are identical, and one of them is already suffering from the symptoms of ADHD, the chances of the other child also developing the problem are about 83%. The overall percentage falls down to 39% if the twins are fraternal. All of these statistics can easily show the close link of ADHD with genetics.

Anatomy of The Brain

More research is being carried out to find out the relation between the structure of the brain and ADHD. It has already been figured out that there are some parts of the brain in kids that do not tend to develop fast in comparison to others. However, having this said, it does not indicate that kids suffering from symptoms of ADHD are not talented or not smart. To put it in simple words, some parts of the brain take some more amount of time to get developed fully. Some of such structures play an essential role in relation to emotional control and working memory. That is the primary reason why the brain system of self-management suffers. However, by the time the affected child reaches adulthood, all these important structures undergo change and tend to attain the completely developed stage.

You will have to properly understand that the way the brain functions can be compared to the shifting of gears. All the related parts need to work together to write or read. The structures that play the role of connecting the various brain cells are the neurons. When a child suffers from the symptoms of ADHD, all these neural networks take more time to get developed. One of such neural networks serves the purpose of making the child get into a resting phase. It is often referred to as the 'default mode network.' When a child suffers from this disorder, they fail to concentrate properly as this default mode network takes more time in putting other aspects to hold or rest. Another important pathway that gets affected is the frontoparietal network. It is the network that serves the purpose of a child's ability to get to know and learn to brand new things and also make essential decisions.

Other Related Factors

In some of the cases, children might develop ADHD when the child experiences some sort of head injury during their childhood days. Some types of parental exposure might also turn out to be quite harmful to children and often result in ADHD. Such exposures involve alcohol and nicotine. There are some rare cases where the concerning symptoms of ADHD arise because of environmental reasons. One such example is when a child comes under exposure to lead, and it often results in abnormal behavior and stunted development.

Symptoms of ADHD

As already discussed before, the primary symptoms related to ADHD in a child involve patterns of impulsive and hyperactive behavior. All of them are primarily inattentive. The ADHD symptoms can be seen from childhood. Additionally, the symptoms can be seen from as early as the age of three years. However, in general, the symptoms of the disorder might start showing during any time before the affected child crosses the mark of twelve years.

Let us delve deep into some common symptoms of ADHD.

Hyperactivity and Impulsivity

Does your child like to stay in motion all the time? Does he/she keep talking excessively even when it is not necessary? Well, all of these are the most common symptoms of hyperactivity. Your child is impulsive when you find them continuously interrupting the concerned questioner and just keep answering every question when they are not supposed to. It is also at times when your child cannot just wait for getting or doing anything. All those children who suffer from ADHD have the unavoidable requirement to break through others' conversations, activities, and games. In fact, they start showing problems when they are asked to complete something silently.

Children suffering from ADHD keep fidgeting their hands or feet. Whenever they are asked to sit silently for some time, they keep squirming in their seat. They might even start running or climbing around when you ask them to sit quietly in one place. It might be taken as one of the primary reasons why children with ADHD face a number of problems while attending school. Another very common symptom involves your child being excessively concentrated on his/her requirements or needs that they just ignore or do not pay attention to the needs of others. They might experience continuous turmoil. Also, your child might find it difficult to put some barrier on their emotions. Yes, they might show a lot of interest in various things. However, when it comes to the point of finishing them before opting for the next, they just try to skip that part and leave the task as it is, incomplete.

Inattention

In case you notice that your child is continuously making silly mistakes in their school works or they are not trying to pay enough attention to even the minute things, the chances are high that he/she is inattentive. Some other examples of being inattentive are when your child does not tend to respond in the way they actually should in cases when you are conversing with them directly. Also, your child might showcase signs that they are not at all completely focused on the simplest tasks during the course of the day. Inattention can be figured out in various other forms where the child gets distracted very easily from the task they are doing. They might even suffer a lot with organizational skills. You can easily figure out that your child is suffering from inattention whenever they try to turn away their eyes from activities that need them to stay focused, for instance, school homework. You can also understand the same from various situations where your child makes it a habit to lose essential things that are needed for completing their assignments or some other important matter.

ADHD and Its Types

You can never find one common size that can fit all the concepts of ADHD. It is mainly because that neurodevelopmental disorder tends to take a different shape for different people. Although the majority of the symptoms are more or less the same, the symptoms shown by your child might not be the exact same as those shown by some other child. You will come to know about the various types of ADHD in this section.

Primarily Inattentive ADHD

It is the case when children find it tough to maintain sustained attention. So, they just end up making some silly mistakes. Even when you provide them with a completely detailed token of instructions, they won't be able to follow them properly. Also, they are quite bad at organizing stuff. Regardless of the fact that how insignificant or small the outer stimulus is, children suffering from ADHD of this nature might get distracted very easily.

Primarily Hyper-Active Impulsive Disorder

It can be seen in all those children whose primary problem is that they continuously want to be engaged in movement of some sort. They either keep fidgeting or struggle. They do not want to be seated in one place for a long amount of time. Self-control is something that they can never practice. Children with this type of ADHD often try to blurt out things during the most unfortunate timings or moments.

Combination ADHD

All those children whose symptoms do not completely fall under any of the above-mentioned types are suffering from combination ADHD. It is because they have something from both. In fact, this type of ADHD is regarded as the most common type of ADHD when it comes to children.

Diagnosis of ADHD

Now that you are completely aware of the symptoms, in case you think that your child is also showing some of the signs, the time has come when you might just need to consult with a general physician regarding the same. If you are not sure regarding whether you are opting for the correct steps or not, you might also have some sort of consultation with the teachers of your child. Try to figure out if they also discuss the same kind of symptoms that is displayed by your child in their school. Indeed, your general physician will not be assessing ADHD. However, opting for a general physician first is very important. Your general physician might ask you some common questions during your first visit.

- What are the symptoms that you are recently noticing in your child? From when you have been noticing all these?
- When do you think the symptoms get triggered the most? Is it at home or during school hours?
- Are the symptoms making it tough for him/her to socialize with other people?
- Is there anyone in your family who also has had ADHD?
- Have you noticed some other symptoms other than the ones related to ADHD that you feel are worth noticing?

Right after you are done with your consultation with your general physician, he/she would advise you to keep your child under proper observation for some time. The time span is generally over ten to eleven weeks. During this period, you will come to see whether there is any kind of improvement in your child or not. You will also come to know whether the pre-existing symptoms remain the same or worsen. In some cases, the general physician might also advise you for parent training or some education program that primarily concentrates on ADHD. However, there is something at this point that you will have to understand. When you are advised to opt for parent training, it does not indicate at all that it is all because of you or you are a bad parent.

It is aimed at teaching you all those methods with which you can easily tackle your child in a better way and also bring about some improvement in their present condition. After this time span, if you still find that the symptoms haven't improved, you will need to opt for a formal assessment with the help of a specialist. In case you think about what nature of specialist you will be referred to, there are quite a few of them who can help you with your concern. You might be asked to consult any of them-

- When it is about child health, you might be recommended to visit a pediatrician
- A child psychiatrist relying on the patient's age
- A social worker, occupational therapist, or a specialist in learning disability

The person, whom you are being referred, will vary depending on your location along with the age of the patient. Whether your child is actually suffering from problems of ADHD can never be determined by a single test. However, a detailed kind of assessment by an expert for this matter can definitely throw some light upon the real matter. Some of the common aspects of such assessments involve-

- A range of interviews with your child and you
- A physical examination of the affected child can be brought to light then

- Interviews of some other individuals are also carried out, such as family members, partners, and teachers.

However, to properly diagnose a teenager or a child with problems of ADHD, there are some fixed criteria that require to be followed.

- The symptoms have started showing themselves right before the child touches the mark of 12 years.
- The symptoms can be seen and are consistent for a minimum of six months.
- The symptoms are making it really hard for the affected child to live a normal life both at social and academic levels.
- The symptoms should not be showcasing themselves only in one place, however, under two completely different settings. For example, at home and also at school, so that the symptoms shown by the affected child are not a result of the teacher's treatment or parental control.

ADHD and Its Treatments

If you are looking out for ways to improve the condition of your child and if you want them to live a normal and happy life without losing his/her momentum during any daily activities, then you will have to seek the help of treatment. You will get the option of opting for medication or therapy. However, to get better results, it is always suggested to maintain a proper balance of the two.

Medication

To treat ADHD, you will get a total of five types of medicines that can be used under license. However, right before we can move forward with discussing all these medications, you will have to keep in mind that you can never get any kind of permanent cure for ADHD. So, it can be said that even if you opt for medication, your child will get only some temporary kind of relief from all the symptoms. He/she will regain the capability to again practice new skills, have a calmer demeanor, and also some brand new skills. Some types of medications can only be administered after some intervals. Also, there are the ones that you will give to your child on a regular basis.

Regardless of the medication type that is administered to a child, they will never be provided with any kind of big doses at the starting for the sake of their safety. To properly administer the effects of the medications on your child and also to get him/her used to them, small doses will be suggested. With passing time, the doses can be either be decreased or increased gradually if something of this sort is necessary. Also, you will have to take your child for regular checkups to the concerned specialist so that regular monitoring can be performed. The specialist will also tell you after some time whether the prescribed medications or dosage are actually helping your child or not. If you figure out some sort of side effects on your child related to the medications, never hesitate to bring the same to the attention of the specialist. Some of the common medications that are used for ADHD treatment are:

- **Dexamfetamine:** The medication can be provided to any person who is above the mark of five years of age. It is consumed as a tablet. In some cases, this medication might be prescribed two times a day. In general, it is administered once every day. However, this medication might also result in some sort of side effects such as a reduction in appetite, mood swings, dizziness, and headaches, among various others.

- **Methylphenidate:** You can regard this medication as the most common and most widely used one for treating ADHD. The primary reason that can be found behind the popularity of this medication is that it can be provided to anyone, no matter it is a teenager, children, or an adult. One thing that you will have to keep in mind that the age of the person needs to be above five years. Some of the common side effects of this medication include an increase in the level of blood pressure along with heart rate, stomach aches, and also lack of sleep.

- **Guanfacine:** The medication comes with the power of reducing blood pressure and also helps in improving attentive power. It is meant for kids right above the age mark of 5 years. The medication is not meant for adults.

Therapy
Another option that you can choose is therapy. There are various types of therapies that you can easily select from. Let us have a look at them.

- **Psychoeducation:** It is a therapy session where your child and you will have to speak up about ADHD and also gain knowledge about the various side-effects. Therapy of this sort helps in making it easier to diagnose and also understand ADHD symptoms.

- **Behavior therapy:** In this type of therapy, not only the suffering kid is involved but also their parents and teachers. A proper system is developed in which the related child will get some kind of reward for showing good behavior. Any sort of behavior that you desire your child to develop can be easily inculcated with the help of this method.

- **Social skills training:** In this nature of therapy, the concept of role-playing is put into use to help the child learn how to socialize with others. They also come to know about certain behaviors that they should opt for when in a public setting.

- **Parent training:** Programs of this type are meant specifically for the parents in order to make them aware of some new techniques with which they can easily improve the symptoms of their child. Mostly group programs are used for this where parents can discuss with the parents of other children about the problems of their children.

Chapter 2: Common Myths About ADHD

Misconceptions and myths can be found in every minute portion of life, and thus ADHD is no different. However, when myths and misconceptions start forming deeper roots in society, it can make the whole situation turn into some major problem. People start believing them, and the ultimate result is that you won't be able to differentiate between true and false. That is the primary reason why misconceptions and myths regarding any kind of disease can result in serious harm. So, it is essential to debunk such myths and just see the problem in the real light. Also, myths and misconceptions can sometimes make the treatment procedure quite tiresome. We will debunk some of the primary myths about ADHD in this chapter so that you do not end up misunderstanding your child.

ADHD Cannot Be Regarded As a Real Disorder

ADHD has always been recognized as a serious disorder by most medical professionals, psychological and psychiatric experts, and organizations and associations in the United States. Some of the major organizations are APA or American Psychiatric Association, NIH or National Institute of Health, along with the

Center for Disease Control and Prevention. One of the primary factors that actually contribute to myths or misunderstandings about the status of ADHD is that there is a lack of any proper test that can truly identify the disorder. Just like other serious medical conditions, a medical expert or a doctor cannot just confirm the diagnosis of ADHD with the help of imaging and laboratory test. Indeed there is no proper test for the diagnosis of ADHD; there are certain specific and clear criteria that require to be met for the diagnosis. Mental health professionals and doctors can put into use these criteria, along with detailed history and information regarding the concerned person's behaviors, to provide a reliable diagnosis.

Another important factor is that the symptoms of ADHD are not always defined clearly. ADHD exists on a proper sequence of behaviors. All of us experience some sort of problems regarding focusing and attention at times. However, for a person who is suffering from ADHD, all these symptoms might turn out to be severe enough that they can easily hamper their daily functioning. ADHD symptoms might also resemble some other conditions. Undiagnosed or pre-existing medical problems need to be recognized before the diagnosis of ADHD.

ADHD Is Often Over-Diagnosed

The evidence regarding this is kind of mixed. According to annual data, there is an increase in the diagnosis of ADHD in children in the U.S. But the reports also state that the rates of other serious conditions, like anxiety, depression, and autism, have also shown an increase. Talking about ADHD in specific, various studies have demonstrated that the condition might get under-diagnosed in certain cases where the overall symptoms are much less noticeable. A prominent example gathered from the pieces of evidence shows that ADHD might manifest in a different way in female children. While female children suffering from ADHD have fewer chances of showing any kind of hyperactive symptoms, they might still have some impairment of significant kind with focus and mental tasks. A wide range of studies has suggested that female children are less likely to get diagnosed and also receive any kind of treatment related to ADHD than male children.

Some other studies suggest that ADHD is most of the time over-diagnosed, however, particularly in boys. Increased rates of ADHD in male children might be partly because of the stereotypes regarding male behavior; for instance, boys tend to act out physically. Boys might also be more likely to show disruptive and ADHD symptoms, which directly enhances the chances that teachers, parents, and also doctors will notice all their behaviors. It has been found that ethnic, socioeconomic, and racial factors also play some role in the disparity in the treatment and diagnosis of ADHD. In accordance to a study from the year 2016, white children were most likely to be diagnosed with ADHD and also receive treatment for the same. Although the researchers find these findings to imply over-diagnosis, they suggest that under-treatment and under-diagnosis of Latino and African American children with ADHD could be a more specific interpretation of the gathered data.

Another research proposed that ADHD in adults is also over-diagnosed. It is often suggested that adults might get diagnosed with the symptoms of ADHD because of the medicalization of their typical personality variations and life experiences. In some of the cases, other types of learning disabilities or mental health conditions are often misdiagnosed as the symptoms of ADHD. The primary risk involved with the over-diagnosis of ADHD is unnecessary treatment along with stimulant medication. Although the related drugs can work as an effective treatment for ADHD, when provided to someone who does not require them, they might be misused.

ADHD Can Only Be Found In Children

The ADHD symptoms require to be present by the age mark of seven years to properly meet the criteria of diagnosis. However, there are people who often remain undiagnosed until they reach adulthood. It not at all uncommon for some parents to get diagnosed with ADHD along with their children at the same point in time. As any adult starts learning in detail about the actual condition, they might start recognizing the traits of ADHD along with the related behaviors in themselves. While thinking about their childhood, they might just realize that the struggles they faced at school were most probably the result of problems related to attention that went untreated or unnoticed. For children and parents, proper diagnosis at any point might seem like a relief. Getting the ability to put the symptoms under some kind of names while also knowing that there are ways to properly manage them might be reassuring.

A lot of children, who get diagnosed with the symptoms of ADHD, might continue to showcase the symptoms even as teens and adults. However, the overall nature of the symptoms might change as they grow. For instance, the hyperactive nature of behaviors that are common in kids has the tendency to reduce with age. However, distractibility, inattention, and restlessness might persist into their adulthood. ADHD in adults, which is managed poorly, might often result in chronic problems in relationships and at work. Untreated and undiagnosed ADHD can also be linked with substance misuse, depression, and anxiety.

ADHD Is the Result of Bad Parenting

Parents of ADHD children might often worry that they are the ones to be blamed for the behaviors of their children. However, the overall condition is not caused by bad parenting strictly. Any child, no matter they are suffering from the symptoms of ADHD or not, can get affected adversely by critical and punitive parenting or a chaotic home. All such factors might make the whole situation tougher for the children to cope with the problems of ADHD; however, they are not the primary cause of the condition. With that said, parents might want to consider adapting their style of parenting to support their ADHD child in a better way. It has been found that children suffering from ADHD tend to benefit from consistent and clear consequences and expectations, along with having some predictable nature of routine at their home.

One of the Surest Symptoms of ADHD Is Hyperactivity

The 'attention deficit' portion of the name has resulted in misunderstandings regarding the overall nature of the condition and has also perpetuated various myths regarding the symptoms. In fact, there are various ADHD types that we have already discussed in the previous chapter. Hyperactive behaviors can be found only in the predominantly hyperactive-impulsive type and cannot be found in the predominantly inattentive one. In order to reduce any kind of confusion, ADHD of the predominantly inattentive nature is often referred to as attention-deficit disorder or ADD. Any individual who showcases inattentive symptoms might appear easily distracted and daydreamy. They might also be careless, forgetful, and disorganized. ADHD of this type is overlooked most of the time. It is mainly because it is of a less disruptive nature than the hyperactive one. But the related symptoms can still be dreadful to the one who is experiencing all of them.

While any child suffering from ADHD would not outgrow the disorder typically, sometimes adults report growing out of the behaviors of hyperactive nature that they had in their childhood. In some cases, hyperactivity might get replaced by apathy and restlessness.

People Suffering From ADHD Cannot Focus At All

Provided the name of the condition, it might be really confusing for some people to see someone with ADHD/ADD intently focusing on any activity. It will be more accurate to describe the portion of 'attention-deficit' as difficulty in regulating concentration in place of the ability to pay any attention. Although individuals suffering from ADHD face difficulty organizing, completing, and focusing on tasks, it is not at all uncommon for them to get absorbed in all those activities that they find interest in. In fact, hyperfocus of such a sustained level can indicate when someone has ADHD.

Stimulants Might Result in Addiction and Drug Abuse

There is a major concern that the stimulant medications that are used for treating problems of ADHD can result in substance misuse. But it has been found from researches that ADHD, when left untreated, can easily enhance the risk of a person for the disorder of substance use. Depression or anxiety can also result from untreated ADHD. An individual might misuse illicit and licit drugs in order to medicate their symptoms of ADHD along with any other secondary nature of the psychological condition. It has also been found that all those who receive proper treatment for ADHD come with a lower percentage of substance misuse, along with stimulant medication.

Medication Can Completely Treat ADHD

Medication cannot cure the symptoms of ADHD. However, it can readily help in managing the symptoms when administered under the guidance of mental health professional. ADHD can be regarded as a lifelong and chronic condition. If someone gets prescribed to have ADHD medication during their childhood, they might have to continue consumption of the same as an adult as well. People might just carry on with the same symptoms as adults that they had as children. The symptoms might also lessen or just change with time. Developmental alterations in the brain can explain all such changes partly. However, they might also be the reflection of the ways someone has gained knowledge about coping.

Individuals suffering from ADHD might often develop organizational skills and coping strategies to help them move on with the condition. They can just expand and continue to build up all these skills all throughout the course of their lives. They might also decide to pair the same along with medications.

ADHD Develops When Children Are Lazy

It can be regarded as a proper way of demeaning the actual problem as ADHD is not a result of a lack of motivation or laziness. It is an actual medical problem that needs to be addressed properly. When your child is suffering from the symptoms of ADHD, it is not the case that he/she is not trying to focus on things. In actuality, they are giving their best to do so. However, they cannot end up doing so. In case you are just asking your child to concentrate more and being rude/angry on the, as they are not trying, it is actually worthless. It is similar to getting angry at someone as they cannot see something, while in reality, they are actually blind. Your child's attitude is not the main factor that is trying to affect the child's attentive power. It is only because of some physical differences that exist in their brain for which they cannot do or see things like any other child. Expecting them to perform or behave like the rest of the children when they are not even built in that way is foolish.

In fact, there are cases where people do not even clearly understand the concept of ADHD and blame their children for not focusing on something or behaving a particular way. All of this indirectly worsens the symptoms of the child and also makes him/her feel guilty. When your child is suffering from the problems of ADHD, you will have to develop a huge number of reminders to make them actually do some task. However, that does not indicate that your child is lazy. All it means is that they do not possess the brain structure to dedicate so much effort. Even playing a very easy game of building blocks might turn out to be mentally tiring for a child who is suffering from the symptoms of ADHD. So, it will be better for them if you can just stop judging them or comparing them for staying behind other children.

Myths and misconceptions regarding ADHD might turn out to be harmful at many levels. Myths can make timely diagnosis a difficult job. Understanding and awareness of ADHD can help a lot in combating various kinds of challenges that are faced by the sufferers of the same.

Chapter 3: Opting for Self-Care

The primary step that is needed to start dealing with the problems of ADHD is to let your child know how they can take care of themselves. As responsible parents, you will surely take good care of your child. However, when your child gets some idea of taking care of themselves, nothing can actually be better than that as they will know how to be self-reliant. Additionally, all those children who are suffering from the problems of ADHD also get to learn to follow through and just stay on track. It is quite essential to teach your children not to rely on the verbal instructions from your side alone but also to do certain things by themselves. All of this will provide them with the needed help to gain autonomy. No matter what happens in life, getting indulged in self-care is very important.

A very common example is to teach your child the way they can properly listen to an alarm clock while waking up and not just rely on their mother's voice. However, you will also have to show your love along with faith in your children and just them they are worth believing in. Regardless of what happens, you just can never give up on your child. Whether it is about applying toothpaste on their toothbrush or as simple as pouring their juice in their own glass, every minute task can be succeeded if they get the correct support. The scale of your child, along with their background of accountability, might not match with that of other children who are of his/her age, and that is completely okay. It is often said that children suffering from the problems of ADHD are generally behind other children in their daily activities by almost 30%, and their skills of self-management take the hit.

Thus, if you are want to make your child learn about the various to get active in self-care, there are some strategies that you will have to follow.

Concentrating on the Related Advantages

It is quite a common thing that while talking about self-care, some sort of luxurious thoughts might pile up inside your mind. However, that is not exactly what self-care is about. It comes with the benefit of being practiced in your own way. It might also be a proper set of some practical actions, tailored especially for the health of your child who is suffering from the symptoms of ADHD. In case you want to provide your child with the best selfocare possible, you will have to first urge them to find out what they actually want. Whenever children suffering from ADHD are not stressed to engage in self-care or just look after themselves, they tend to become more depleted emotionally, depressed, more exhausted, and even more angry. As you make your child understand how they can put themselves on the first position of their priority list, they will just stop feeling undeserving and overwhelmed.

Indeed, at times, your child who is a teenager might just feel that they can start looking after their own selves after every problem gets sorted. However, that might just turn into a far-fetched dream. You will have to first put yourself in the first place and just make your child do the same. If you start by asking your children to have some thoughts about self-care, the chances of them getting uncomfortable are quite high. So, there is no requirement to rush with the same. Just try to take it forward with one action at a time. Keep teaching them minute actions, all of which collectively can help in making them feel a lot better.

However, there are many cases where the concerned children tend to move farther from their parents as they were asked to be self-sustainable. It is primarily because children suffering from the symptoms of ADHD always require someone by their side. As you ask them to suddenly start learning to do things on their own, they just fear abandonment. They have always got the risk of rejection in their minds that might turn out to be quite toxic. It might also stop them from getting adapted to a self-sustainable lifestyle. If you ever notice all such things in your suffering child as well, it will be better for you to opt for a completely different approach. You can start asking him/her various questions like – "Do you feel that I will love you any less in case you start taking care of your own self?" You will have to make your suffering child realize that all that you want them is to develop more in life. Make them realize that you are urging them for self-care for their own good.

A great thing that can be done on your part is to make your child realize the various advantages of self-care or self-reliance. Provide them with certain examples, such as – as they become self-reliant, they will get the chance to visit various places, or they will be able to complete their own tasks even at times when someone is not present around them to provide them with the needed help. The primary idea is that you will need to make your suffering child realize that there is more good in being self-reliant than the worse or bad. Make sure you are careful with the tone of your voice, along with the usage of words. It is because a child suffering from ADHD might get affected quite easily.

After you are done with saying all your things, try to figure out the way in which your child reacts. You will have to find out whether the reaction is negative or positive. In case it is positive, you will come to know that you are doing everything in the perfect way. You might also maintain a note on the willingness of your child to be self-reliant, along with the self-growth shown by them every day. It will help you to keep a proper track of your road to progress in teaching your child self-care.

Teaching Your Child to Follow Through on Their Commitments

Whenever you try to help your child suffering from ADHD with even the smallest job, you will be saving a great amount of time on your part. You will also be able to make your child feel that they are very important to you. However, are you actually helping them to grow in the future? Children suffering from ADHD find it very difficult to follow through with anything, be it instructions or commitments. There are some ways in which you can easily make your child aware of the concept of commitment without even triggering the symptoms.

Working on Skills of Organization

One of the primary challenges that are faced by the parents of every ADHD child is to teach their child how to effectively follow through. The main reason behind this is the low level of presence of organizational skills in children suffering from ADHD. You can also consider this as the main reason why they always forget all kinds of obligations that they have. However, there are also various cases where the parents themselves promote their children unknowingly to just use ADHD as a form of excuse to turn away from almost every vital thing in their lives. Only because a child is suffering from the symptoms of ADHD does not indicate that they do not possess what is needed to be productive. They can also wake up in the morning and spend their day according to a routine like everyone else. All that you will need to do is to just teach all of that in the proper way.

One of such strategies is to take the help of a planner that can aid your child brush up on their skills of organization. As you teach your child the way a planner is put into use, you will also have to make them understand how they can properly map out all their tasks in the same. Try to teach your child to prepare his/her own routine. For instance, just consider that your child has several assignments to be submitted at school in the coming weeks. You will have to tell your child to make the possible entries of the assignments in his/her planner so that they can easily keep track of all those things that they will have to get done within a specific deadline. However, noting down all their deadlines along with to-do lists is not the only thing that they should do. They will have to do a lot more work. After your child has properly set up the deadline, it is your duty now as a parent to make your child understand the usage of a planner in the first place.

It is your duty to teach your child how to properly break one assignment into various parts and just focus on one single part at a time. The small parts have to be treated as the stepping stones for reaching their final goal. In the same way, if any examinations are coming up in your child's school, you will have to teach your child how to prepare a proper study plan to get done with everything on time right before their exams. Make your child properly understand the importance of keeping something in their planner as the daily goal, regardless of how big or small it is. Teach your child how to find out their strategies for attaining their goal. In this very way, steadily and slowly, you can make your child invested in his/her studies completely.

Implementation of Pets to Teach Responsibility

When your child is suffering from the symptoms of ADHD, pets can actually have some great effects on them. Pets can be used to breed in the sense of responsibility and routine for the child. It is primarily because pets can bring in a huge bunch of positivity at once. Ask your child what they want and get them that, be it a rabbit, dog, cat, or some other pet. No matter what the pet is, you will have to provide your child with the duty and responsibility to feed his/her pet and also take them out for walks if needed. Your ADHD child will give their best to take care of their pet as they love the animal. Also, taking proper care of a pet will also provide them with a great amount of love in return. Getting a pet like a dog or even a cat is always better as even if your kid just forgets to feed them on time, the pet will try to remind them of the same in some way or the other to feed them. Animals come with their ways to make people understand things. Also, gifting a pet to your child will make them feel quite responsible. At times, a little bit of push or motivation is all that is needed by a student to get going.

Practicing Color Coding

A great strategy that can be put to use to help your child who is suffering from ADHD on their organizational skills is color-coding. Indeed, children suffering from the symptoms of ADHD will surely face some academic challenges. However, that does not provide them with any kind of excuse to give up on stuff. Color coding is a strategy that can help anyone suffering from ADHD to learn various things within a short time. You can help your child by separating various subjects in the planner using different colors. It will help your child understand stuff by only having a look at the planner. For instance, if your child has mathematics homework, assign a color, suppose yellow, for the subject. Make sure that your child puts some yellow-colored labels where they will be doing the homework. You can also make your child wear a yellow bracelet so that they can be aware of the mathematics homework.

Using the strategy of the bracelet can help a lot as it can serve the purpose of being a visual reminder of any kind of task. After the homework gets checked by the teacher, there is no need to wear the bracelet anymore. In case you are willing to take things a little further, then you can opt for making folders for each of your child's subject and just label them in specific colors. Organizational skills can be made quite strong with the help of color-coding. It is a strategy that can be followed by your child easily.

Helping Your Child to Prepare Routines

You can never find an imperfect or perfect way to raise a kid who is suffering from the symptoms of ADHD. However, one thing that is quite essential when it comes to proper parenting is to instill a properly structured environment for the child. It also includes introducing the child to the concept of routine. Whenever this concept comes up, a very common question will surely develop in your mind – "How a proper structure can help my kid?" Well, we will be discussing everything about this in this section.

What Is the Importance of Routine?

Whenever there is a discussion regarding the perfect way of bringing up a child suffering from ADHD, you will surely come across the term 'structure.' What does the term refer to? It is a kind of environment that is more organized and predictable. To properly bring in structure in the life of your child, you will have to design a proper schedule for them along with routines for day-to-day life. It is quite essential for your child to properly understand the expectations, consequences, and rules so that their life environment is predictable. All of this can help them in getting the feeling of security. The capability of regulation is something that children with ADHD do not possess. They have to face a lot of distractions and so staying focused on any specific thing turns out to be nearly impossible for them.

Self-control is a huge issue for all those children who are suffering from the symptoms of ADHD. We will discuss more about the same in the upcoming chapters. In this section, we will only talk about the basics of routine, the importance of the same, and how to properly set them. When there is a fixed routine present, completing even the toughest jobs will not feel like a burden for a kid. They will slowly learn how they can fix some time for simple things like brushing their teeth, taking a shower, or even finishing their homework. To put it in simple words, with the help of routines, you will get the chance to teach some great habits to your child.

How Can a Routine Be Developed?

An essential thing about all of this is how to develop a proper routine for your child? If you are feeling confused, then there is nothing to worry about, as I have provided some essential points below t get this done properly.

- The first thing that you will have to take care of is to make sure that the instructions provided by you are to the point and clear. In case you want your child to clean up his/her room, do not provide them with instructions such as – "Go and clean the room." You will have to be specific regarding what you want them to do. For instance, "Put the toys in the cupboard and the books on the shelf." Your instructions need to be specific like this. Children suffering from ADHD need to be told what you are expecting from them exactly, and then only they can work on the same.

- It is also quite essential for you to only assign all those jobs/tasks to your child that you surely know he/she can do on their own. As they succeed in one of the tasks, it can promote them to the next level to opt for other things. In short, they can start developing a lot of confidence. On the contrary, if you only try to provide them with tasks that they cannot do on their own, it will only end up demotivating them. The only aim is to develop a proper routine and encourage your child to get their tasks done on their own.

- It would be better if you can write down the routines on behalf of your child. No task can be clumped with each other. It requires to be written in a proper sequence. Each of the sequences should only have two to five tasks. If you fail to do so, your child will end up getting confused. Try to place the routine at a place that can be noticed easily by your child. A properly written set of tasks or instructions are always considered better for children suffering from ADHD as they might just forget the verbal instructions very easily. If your child has to get done with a larger task, you will have to break the same into various small steps. It will make sure that your child continues on track.

- Never try to give less importance to physical activities. Make sure that you include some kind of physical activity in their routine. It is essential for the betterment of your child's physical and mental fitness. For all those children who are suffering from the symptoms of ADHD, physical activities might turn out to be quite stimulating. In fact, it is advised by specialists and doctors to opt for physical activities.

- A great way to make sure that the system of schedule and routine works in a superb way for your child is to develop a proper set of rules for getting rewards. As your child gets done with a task as you asked them to do, you will have to provide them with a reward as you have set.

- At times, the efforts from the side of your child might not show any results. That is completely fine. You will have to acknowledge the fact that he/she is trying their best to improve. The reward for proper behavior needs to be frequent in comparison to punishment for doing something bad.

- It will be foolish of you if you want your child to showcase great improvements immediately. You will have to provide the proper time to get themselves accustomed. They will literally have to discard their old habits and develop new ones. All of this cannot happen overnight. So, it will be better for you and your child to expect gradual improvements and not immediate ones.

- Lastly, do not try to crowd their routine excessively. You will have to leave some free time in the routine where your child can spend some time on their own. All of us need our very own downtime. So, it is quite essential to schedule some amount of free time.

Assisting Them to Deal With Difficulties While Dressing Up

The complete act or task of putting on clothes might turn out to be a difficult task for a child who is suffering from the symptoms of ADHD. However, you can easily make the whole task an easy one by taking into account some easy steps. Some children might face a problem with the fabric type that the clothes are made of, or some might just forget the proper sequence in which they are meant to put on the clothes. The nature of problems will vary from one child to another.

- The primary thing that you will have to do is to calm down your child. N case your child needs to bathe in the morning, you will have to dry him/her off with the help of a heavily textured towel. According to some studies, using textured towels can help in calming down the brains of all those children who are suffering from ADHD. It will help in dressing them up as an easy task. It will also provide your child with tactile stimulation.

- You will come to see that your ADHD child often complains about the ways their clothes are. They might find their clothes itchy all the time. However, parents tend to overlook their complaints at times and do not believe them. Make sure you never turn your face from such issues. Whenever your child says that the clothing is not comfortable, just believe them. Try to opt for clothes made of those fabrics that you think your child is fond of. Also, ensure that the clothes that you make them wear do not have any kind of labels or tags that might result in irritation.

- There are cases where children with ADHD tend to feel more secure when they opt for tight-fitted underwear. If that is the case with your own child, try to opt for all those underwear that comes with snug-fitting, such as performance apparel. However, you will also have to make sure that the fabrics are breathable and of high quality so that it does not make the clothing uncomfortable for your child.

- Try to keep the clothing simple. That is the reason why pants with waistbands that comes with the ease of being pulled up are more advised than pants with zippers or buttons. Also, you can opt for giving your child lessons on dressing, like how they can tie their shoelaces or how to button their shirt during free time.

- Always try to keep the wardrobe of your child as simple as possible. Do not just leave it overflowing or untidy. It might result in making your child confused as to what to wear or where a specific pant or shirt is. You can opt for categorization of their closet so that they can get what they want easily.

Chapter 4: ADHD Reinforcements

We will talk about the essential reinforcements related to ADHD that can help in the improvement of the symptoms of your child. Children suffering from ADHD are always in need of proper support. All that they want is to take the support of others. As they get proper attention from their caregivers, it helps in making them feel soothing besides making them feel better. When ADHD children grow up, everyone around them, including their parents, expect them to abide by some rules and also take care of themselves. Providing an ADHD child with various types of restrictions will never help in solving the problem. You will have to understand all those actions that can help in benefitting your child and also improve their overall behavior. You will have to be aware of all those actions that can actually make their condition worse. As you have proper knowledge of these, along with the reinforcements of the various negative effects of ADHD, you will get the power to reduce all those things.

The primary reinforcements of ADHD have been properly discussed in this section, which might, at times, work in unison along with other types of behaviors to make the symptoms of your child worse.

Accommodation

In most cases, a child will not showcase vigorous behaviors related to ADHD as long as you say 'yes' to them. It is quite normal for the caregivers of the child to provide them with support and comfort the very moment as the child starts whining or creates problems. All such things tend to happen when your child starts showcasing anxiety symptoms, displaying rage, being excessively self-critical or overreacting. Every time a child in any family gets diagnosed with the symptoms of ADHD, the adults of the family try to provide all sort of support to the child. Accommodating an ADHD child might also result in a range of problems.

For instance, when your child is acting out and demanding something so that they can soothe their discomfort, you try to bring that exact thing for him/her. In fact, you will bring the same in large quantities so that he/she does not face the discomfort of any kind. All of this will make your child understand that no matter when they display bad behavior, they will get some stuff that they demand. The symptoms of ADHD have a tendency to flare up as you keep doing more for the betterment of your child and also put in a lot of effort.

Let us have a look at one more common example so that you can understand the problem clearly. When your child is not trying to pay any kind of attention to anything, such as at school or at home, he/she might ask you to properly explain the related matter to them as they were inattentive. Right in this way, they will continue depending on you. The end result of this is that they won't be able to learn self-care for fulfilling their own needs or desires. In case you fail to get your child out of this ADHD cycle and toxic behavior, they might not be able to see progress in any part of their life. The teachers in school will never try to help every student speed up. So, you will have to breed in the values of self-care within your child.

In some cases, a child suffering from ADHD might start correlating rescue with love. It is mainly because whenever they find themselves in some sort of difficult phase or dangerous circumstance in life, you will always try to provide them with the required help and get them out of the situation. However, acts of this kind will make your child feel that if they put themselves in difficult situations, they will be getting all sorts of love from you and thus also be valuable. When an ADHD child is accommodated, you will find that they will keep bombarding you with a series of questions that they either know how to solve or know the answer to. Do you have any idea why? It is primarily because parents always try to leave behind all other important things to answer the questions of their child, and children suffering from ADHD actually prefer this. They intentionally want that you do this for them.

Thus, they might try to play dumb or stupid when in actual they are not.

The behavior of this kind often results in assistance from the side of parents as they are aware of not enforcing any kind of conditions on their child or just make them feel accountable. It is your responsibility to provide all sorts of help to your child to overcome their trials. Whenever they are not effective at something, you will have to be there to help them out. Also, your ADHD child might start complaining regarding you not telling them everything. The only reason you are not trying to do so is that you know he/she is not much qualified for all such things. However, things of this sort can easily trigger the symptoms and make them worse.

A self-gratification attitude of toxic nature tends to develop when you start attending to all the needs and worries of your child, even when there is a need to surrender your well-being. In such a case, an ADHD child needs to be pampered at every level. So, they can never come to know about the needs or desires of others. In case you try to accommodate your child, who is suffering from ADHD excessively, along with easements at every single turn to make them achieve their goals, it will result in back lashing later on. So, from the examples and explanations mentioned above, you must have understood that fighting the symptoms of ADHD won't be easy if you just try to accommodate your ADHD child more than the requirement. Let us have a look at some possible reasons behind the habits of over accommodation of parents.

- The most common reason why parents try to over accommodate their child is that they feel if nothing is done from their side, their child might face danger. So, the parents of ADHD children always give their best to opt for the safe route as they do not want their suffering child to get hurt in any possible way. They are aware of the potential risks. So, they do not want their kids to get exposed to the same.

- Another possible reason is that as shame comes in the way of things, parents can compromise everything very easily. Let me explain this to you with the help of an example. Suppose a couple got divorced and the single mother comes to know that her child is suffering from the symptoms of ADHD. The very next moment, she puts herself in a lot of guilt and shame as she starts blaming herself. She thinks that ADHD came into the picture because of negligence on her part. All of this results in over-accommodating the child in every possible sphere of life. The single mother might also blame herself for being busy with work too much and being unable to take care of her child. However, as we have already debunked this myth, we are not delving into the details again. But always make yourself aware that ADHD never results from bad parenting. It comes with various medical reasons behind it.

- A very common reason behind the overaccommodation of a child is that the parents might have faced excessive poverty during their childhood. So, when they have a child of their own now, they would not want the child to face the same. So, they try their best to take care of their child in every possible situation and, at times, in a way that can be considered as more than necessary.

- The next possible reason might be trauma. Parents try to put in efforts to solve every problem that their child might be facing after trauma. They do so to support their child and so that they do not have to deal with threats of any kind themselves. However, while doing so, they just end up over-accommodating their child.

- There are parents who opt for over-accommodation as they do not possess enough time which they can dedicate to their child and help them learn something new on their own. So, they just give in to over-accommodation. They might always be busy because of their schedule at work or because they need to handle a lot of burdens of the family.

So, regardless of the cause of over-accommodation, it is never going to help your child in any possible way. In fact, it might end up hampering the skills of self-management. As a parent, it is quite natural for you to try and make your child's life as easy as possible. However, you will also have to understand that learning to solve problems on your own is a skill that every child requires to progress in life. Just try to think practically. You will not be with your child for your whole life to look after him/her. Indeed, as you help out your child, you will get the chance to develop a new and stronger bond. At the same time, you will be pushing them in the direction of a situation where they might not be able to finish the simplest tasks in life without feedback from your side.

As parents, you will always get a feeling of peace knowing that your child is completely safe with you. However, you will also have to prepare him/her for all those times when you will not be there by their side. So, they will have to learn how to be self-reliant. For example, your child has to complete some project at school, and you are giving your best efforts to make everything simplified for him/her. But you are not actually helping in real. Children need to learn to exert their own selves. Whenever you try to get their tasks done on your own, your child will try to hide behind the same. He/she will never be able to do anything on their own.

When you just keep reminding your child of all those things that need to take or even take all their things yourself so that he/she does not forget them, your child will lose the ability to remember things on their own gradually. It is true that when you try to help your child, it can help in saving a lot of energy and time. In fact, it can also help in simplifying various situations. However, the true fact is that you will not be preparing them for their future. All that you will do is to permit the symptoms of ADHD to sustain.

Attention

The acronym of ADHD is attention deficit hyperactivity disorder. So, the reinforcement that we will discuss in this section is attention. You must have noticed that when you are with your child, and you start conversing with someone affectionately, he/she starts behaving in a furious way. It is mainly because ADHD children tend to feel nervous and threatened when they see their parents sharing any form of an affectionate relationship with someone else other than them. Some of the common actions that can depict this involve your child making weird noises or doing something unacceptable as your attention shifts to someone else. In fact, they might try to target things that are beyond their limits. As your child keeps performing such actions, it is primarily because they want you to attend to them and make you notice what they have actually been up to. At times, you might not even have to talk to someone, but a facial expression of simple nature is enough to trigger such activities.

Indeed, a child tends to get self-centered when they start showcasing ADHD symptoms. If your child starts acting insane, distracting, busy, hyperactive, or annoying, it will not be possible for you to get away from him/her or make the sit quietly in one place. All of this will make your task of completing other chores very tough. One definite thing that can help is flopping your lap by making your child sit and then conversing with someone else.

At school or at home, a child can gather a lot of attention while they perform some off-task activities. In case you find that your child is unable to follow instructions of any kind and is also fiddling most of the time, everyone gets concerned at school. That is the time when the teachers try to get close to your child so that he/she can properly follow the instructions. All of this, in turn, makes your child believe that they have some kind of importance at school and everyone else is always concerned about them. It directs to an opportunity when you can get the chance to motivate your child and also support them. In certain cases, the child might like it when someone pleads to them for giving an answer to some question or also when you keep repeating their name. In this way, they build up the notion that they are very important. Because of the inattentive nature of children suffering from ADHD, they are most of the time asked to sit near or beside the teacher or instructor in public gatherings. Special attention of this nature tends to make them feel good and also helps in the suppression of their symptoms.

You will have to keep in mind and also remind yourself all the time that not every child around you is the same. So, there are some children who are suffering from the symptoms of ADHD and also need a bit more attention and support in comparison to others. Whenever you are in waiting rooms and public places, your child might get out of control and try to gather an audience of his/her own. They might start behaving loudly, without paying any kind of attention to what is being said by you. For instance, suppose you are reading a book while waiting for your train to come, and your ADHD child is sitting right next to you. He/she will continuously try to distract you not for the reason that they are mean but only because they want to spend time with you. In fact, they might try to do something great in order to impress you. However, you can never impose restrictions of any kind on your child, especially in public spaces, as everyone will be staring at you.

Whenever your child keeps making such tantrums for getting attention, there is nothing to worry about that maybe your child does not get enough tantrums. It is mainly because he/she does not have friends of their own. So, they just depend on you entirely. They might even have to go through various jokes and transgressions as they go out.

Avoidance

When adversity is faced, one of the common ways of dealing with various problems is avoidance. As you try to give in to avoidance, it can easily keep up the distractibility and inability to focus going on for a great period of time. The very moment when a child gets diagnosed with the symptoms of ADHD, every individual surrounding the child, along with his/her parents, just gives up on properly understanding anything that is actually going on with their child. It might be either the inability to cooperate or adapt. The primary thing that they can deduce from the whole situation is that there is no need or benefit of talking with their child as their symptoms of ADHD will prevent them from concentrating on the conversation. They just take it for granted that their child will not learn anything ever regardless of how hard they try. That is why they just stop trying.

If the ADHD child fails to respond to something in the way they should and just keeps doing what they are doing, the parents tend to think that is the result of their child's hyper-focusing attitude. It is all that is preventing them from properly listening to the parents. Even when the child lacks courtesy, every individual will just keep saying that it is only because of the symptoms of ADHD that all this is taking place. However, responses of this nature are distractive comments. Sometimes they might benefit your child as they can get the chance to move forward with everything they want to do finally as people will no longer be judging their actions. But when ADHD children come to realize that no one wants to focus on what is being said by them, they just start doing the same without paying attention to what is being said by others. That is the main reason why ADHD children tend to change topics even at times when adults are trying to talk about something important.

It is all because of this kind of distractibility that the suffering child gets the chance to run away from all sorts of assessment, restrictions, and punishment. They just get excessively absorbed in what they are doing. They also stop responding to any external things. In case you try to nag at things, he/she will not even listen to you and instead will turn out to be more lethargic. You might feel that your child is showcasing a distracted attitude, an unfocused nature, and incapability of doing almost anything. However, what actually happens is that the ADHD child tries not to pay any kind of attention to all those things that tend to disrupt them. It is mainly because if they start showcasing all those things, other people will start making them feel that they are nothing but a pure source of disappointment. They would never want to feel that way. So, they just opt for not listening to any nature of negative regarding themselves.

However, if other people can start making the child feel safe and also be appreciative of their qualities, the child will then stop being immersed. He/she will easily open up. Sometimes elders try to brush aside plenty of things by tagging them as impulsive attitude. However, if you just delve in deeper, you will come to know that they are nothing more than avoidance. For instance, if your ADHD child starts being a rebel suddenly by opting for something rash or reckless, you might just think of him/her as being impulsive. However, in actuality, he/she might be just trying to stay away from something or avoid something and simply walk away from any situation. Getting them engaged in any form of impetuous activity, he/she will distract not only others but also their own selves.

Antagonism

The next reinforcement that we will discuss is antagonism. When your ADHD child is upset, there will be times when all they want is to strike back. Generally, children suffering from ADHD are of subtle nature. All that they will do is throw away some household objects or do opt for something very annoying purposefully. However, if you just show exasperation and frustration, your child will slowly learn how to annoy you. The common question that comes to the mind of every parent is that why does the child opt for the antagonism in the first place? The answer to this is various types of relationship issues. In case you want your child to get out of a conflicting cycle, then you will have to start with figuring out some possible ways in which you can handle their antagonism.

A child who is suffering from the symptoms of ADHD is aware all the time of the primary reason that is bothering them. Even when your child is showcasing anger at you, his/her anger might not be because of you but for something completely different that you are not aware of. At times, antagonism takes place as the parents fail to pay attention or just cannot keep up with the request of the children. In case you are trying to find out the reason behind the antagonistic behavior of your child, then let me just remind you that it is not going to be easy at all. It is never that easy to untangle relationships as they are quite complex. It might be because of the existence of certain old incidents or situations that are continuously triggering your child's antagonistic attitude.

Acquisition

At times, certain acts of ADHD children permit them to get fast and easy access to all those things that they want. If the child is showing some sort of reckless behavior and is demanding something from his/her parent, the chances are high that the parents will provide that item to the child. It is mainly because of the impulsive behavior and actions of an ADHD child that you are not aware of what they will do next. They might just start harassing in inappropriate ways or might just pick on other people. All of this provides them with access to all they want as their parents will never want such behavior to continue in a public place. Even the child might just blurt out some statements or words regarding someone that they were never supposed to say. However, they opted for doing so anyway. These are the impulsive actions that you might have to face.

The child enjoys everything that he/she gets from her parents only because of their behavior. However, in the majority of cases, it brings some sort of trouble down the line as well. When problems turn out to be something big in the future, other people have to come into the picture to smoothen out things. As a parent, you will have to keep in mind the number of times your child's rash behavior makes you get into trouble and when some other people have to get in for saving the situation.

With all kinds of trouble between you and your child, you might just wonder whether all of this is doing anything good at all. Well, the benefits that you will receive are the makeups right after the fight. It helps in readily strengthening the bond between you and your child. Indeed, when fights take place, and you overreact, you might feel bad about the same. You might also feel that what you did was not appropriate. However, after that, when you will try to make up for it, you will start feeling good as, without the presence of the fight, you would have never experienced that moment of bonding. Sometimes, you will come to find that your child is not in the mood to forgive you at once, and they need some form of extra effort or pleading. However, he/she will forgive you eventually. It is essential for you to keep an eye on the triggers that push your child in the direction of rough behavior.

The triggers might turn out to be anything – an event that took place in school, something that happened in the earlier days, or even something that was said by you unknowingly. The widely found causes of ADHD involve depleted parents, incompetence insinuations, and inferiority complex.

Chapter 5: Getting Knowledge About Self-Control

One of the things that are common in ADHD children is to act out without thinking properly. You can regard this as one of the reasons why they get into trouble every now and then. Even when you design some rules for them, sometimes they might just lose their control and kick all those rules out of their mind. That is the reason why you will have to continuously work on enhancing the self-control of your child. It can be done easily by going through certain steps that we will discuss in this section. Showcasing some sort of bad behavior will not make your child bad. It is just that they have got some sort of problem with normal behavior.

Helping Them to Connect Behavior With Consequence

Children suffering from ADHD symptoms cannot really delay or inhibit their responses. It can be regarded as a problem that they have to deal with regularly. They always are in the moment, however, not in a good way all the time. At times, they might just act out without providing any form of thought to the situation regarding whether they should have opted for it or not. The primary reason behind this is that they fail to connect their actions with the consequences. When someone has to establish this form of connection, he/she will have to opt for the entire process of pausing and thinking about the events and emotions. They will need to properly weigh the consequences that will follow after they opt for some action and then just make some decision after they are done with considering everything.

Disconnection of this sort between the behavior and consequence is a very common occurrence among all those children who are suffering from the symptoms of ADHD. They are unable to think clearly and might also act out impulsively when things take place all at once. They cannot recall any of the past references that can help in guiding them to make the correct decision. It is the main reason why most ADHD children cannot learn even after they commit their mistake once. They cannot see clearly what is waiting for them ahead in life as they have impairments and problems in their memory. Also, it has been found that the concept of internal language tends to develop at a later phase in the lives of ADHD children. By internal language, I am pointing towards the voice that we all have deep within our minds that helps in guiding us and also regulates all our behaviors.

So, you will need to work as a team with your child and help them in developing some form of connection between all their actions and the related consequences that they might have to face. As they start performing, you will have to provide them with incentives, guidance, cues, and reminders. You will have to teach them to give their best in order to meet the requirements of a specific situation in front of them in place of just acting in an impulsive way. Whenever you find out that your child is not behaving properly, you will have to provide them with your feedback. Try pointing out what is wrong with their behavior and just opt for reinforcement of good behavior. When they start doing something good, motivate them with rewards. It will make your child aware of the nature of the behavior that you want from them.

Setting up a reward system helps in promoting your child towards proper behavior. If they start going off the track, you will have to redirect him/her mildly. Teach your child that right before they decide to respond to something, apply the brakes and try to think whether it is a favorable behavior for the situation. If you can teach all this to your child in the proper way, then you will also have to teach him/her how to be self-aware. Your child will have to be in proper tuning with all those things that are going on. Then only they can successfully connect with the consequences of their actions. For this, he/she will have to be self-aware. It is your duty to design a feedback system of immediate and consistent nature. If you fail to do so, your child will be unable to establish the connection.

Channelizing Your Child's Energy in Productive Things

Children suffering from ADHD often possess a huge amount of energy that they do not even where to channelize. When they cannot figure out the perfect things to spend their energy on, they try to vent out the same at the incorrect places. If you are willing to prevent this from happening, you will have to provide your child with something positive where he/she can vent their energy. That is the reason why doctors and specialists suggest including physical activities in the routines of ADHD children. You might also opt for playing games with your child that would need their energy. Try to design some sort of activity box and just spend some great time with your child. There are various games especially meant for ADHD children that can help in boosting their focus as well.

You can also opt for making a list of chores for your child that they will have to complete. In this way, you can make them busy. Problems regarding self-control also tend to arise when they are at school. You will learn in detail about the same in the upcoming chapters. You must have noticed that whenever you ask your ADHD child to simply wait for something, they tend to have some hard time in waiting for the same. They will easily lose their calm while being agitated. For instance, if you provide them with two options and they have to select one, such as – if they want the larger cookie, they will have to wait for some time but can eat the small one right now, they will opt for the option in which they will not have to wait. However, once you can successfully teach them how to control their energy and breed in patience, everything will turn out to be a lot easier.

Teaching Your Child to Follow Directions

As we already know that children suffering from ADHD find it hard to perform even the most common things in life; one of such things is to follow directions. There are various types of skills that are included in your child following the directions, like staying focused, listening, and also understanding what is being said. All such skills do not develop easily in children suffering from ADHD. If you have seen that when your child is being told to perform multiple tasks at once, and he/she can remember only a few things, you will have to teach them how to properly follow directions in life. Once they can successfully learn this, they will be able to practice self-control as well.

If you want your child to properly comply with the directions provided by you, you will have to make sure first that you have given them the instructions in the right way. In case you have the habit of giving instructions while working, or while chatting with someone else, the chances are high that your child will only hear some parts of the instructions and will understand none. Whenever there is a lot of distraction around them, such as the clanking sound of utensils, water flowing from the tap, or someone else talking, your child will probably think about having ice cream during the summer days. In simple terms, he/she will be lost in their own world of imagination when there are lots of distractions around them while giving instructions.

So, it can be said that drawn-out instructions or directions will not help your child in any way. They will probably find it tough to process everything said by you, especially when you say many things at once. It results in the creation of frustration for both of you. However, in order to make your instructions clear and also help your child understand the same, you will have to follow some very easy steps.

- You will have to start by getting the attention of your child. So, I would suggest you to get close to him/her or maybe just put your hand on his arm or shoulders. You will get the chance to make them stay connected with you in this way.
- Always keep in mind to keep direct eye contact while providing instructions to your child.

- Make sure the directions are simple and actionable. For example, if you just ask them to get ready for their school, they do not have any idea how to do the same. In place of saying that, you will have to provide them with all the related steps – wear fresh underwear, properly put on your shirt, put on your skirt/trouser, and so on.
- Your words need to be clear, and your voice should be firm.
- If you want to explain something to your child, try to do that right before you start giving them instructions. If you opt for explaining something to them after giving the instructions, they will probably just forget what they are supposed to do.
- After you are done with the task of providing all the instructions, stay with them and do not get engaged with your work immediately. Try to stay there for some time and find out whether they are actually attentive and are properly doing what you have asked them to do. If you find your child doing exactly what you have asked them to do, praise him/her immediately so that they can feel motivated. However, if you find out that they are doing it completely wrong, it might be because they haven't understood your instructions clearly. So, do not get anxious and just make them understand the instructions once more.

- If he/she is being stubborn and is not at all complying with the instructions provided by you, you can try to implement some 'If' and 'Then' sentences. Doing so will give them an idea regarding the consequences of their actions. If they agree to comply after this, you must acknowledge them and also praise their efforts. However, if it does not work even after this and does not comply, you will have to opt for a loss of something as its consequence, such as taking away some of their TV time or a favorite toy.
- Your approach needs to be consistent and calm as well. However, if it is only you in the family who is giving in all their efforts in this way, it is not going to work. You will have to talk to your other family members and just make sure that others are following the same way of providing instructions.
- When it comes to daily routines, you can develop a checklist for them to follow. It will not only help them to be on track but will also permit them to work on their own without getting reminded by others to finish their tasks.

Work on Enhancing Your Child's Listening Skills

One of the main reasons why ADHD children tend to react much before thinking properly is that they fail to listen properly. When your child is aware of the right moment to talk, and when they should listen, things will become a lot easier. However, most often, children with ADHD fail to realize the same. It is all that results in problems. You might feel it quite easy for you that the only job is to listen. However, it is not much easy in actuality, especially for ADHD children. It is because to brush up their skills of listening; they will have to wait patiently for their own turn to speak up. But we all know that waiting is a tough job to complete for children with ADHD. There are some ways in which you can provide your child with the required help to work on their listening skills. Let's have a look at them.

- When you are explaining something to your ADHD child, and you are unsure whether he/she is actually listening to you or if they can understand the overall thing or not, you can opt for asking them questions to be sure about the same. Also, make sure you are clear with your instructions, as we have already discussed in the last section. Even when you provide instructions clearly, your child might not be able to understand anything said by you. You can ask him/her to repeat the directions or instructions provided by you. It will help in figuring out whether they understood anything, and if yes, then what. As you provide instructions to your child, keep explaining each instruction or step one after the other. Try not to clump one above the other. You can also opt for using words like first or last so that the instructions seem more structured for your child. It also helps a lot in developing a sense of order.

- Make sure the words used by you are predictable in nature as you talk to your child. Try not to use a lot of new words and give your all to make the conversation predictable. It is essential to enhance the comprehending power of your child in respect to conversations. He/she will know the words that you are going to use, and this, in turn, will make them feel secure and calm.

- Opt for movement as you talk with your child. For instance, you can opt for hand gestures, or you can do something that depicts being in action. All of these strategies have been proven to be helpful when it comes to the context of teaching children with ADHD.

- You can do certain simple things on your part to enhance their skills of listening.

For example, when your child is watching TV, you can just sit beside them and ask him/her to explain to you what just happened on the TV. You will be able to understand whether he/she was actually listening to the TV or not. Whenever your child talks to someone over the phone, you can ask them what did they talk about with the other person right after they hung up the phone.

Instilling Problem Solving Skills

Children suffering from the symptoms of ADHD often lose their calm when they need to solve problems of their daily life. If something seems to be extremely tough for them to deal with, they might even remain stuck with the same for the whole day. They tend to get overwhelmed and also start thinking excessively, which might bring about a sense of uncertainty. In this way, they might be unable to reach any probable conclusion. That is the main reason why they might get frustrated and just act out. In fact, the actual issue tends to get lost among all their confusing and overwhelming thoughts. There are some steps that you will have to teach your child to make their task of problem-solving a lot easier.

- Tell your child to ask themselves what the actual problem is.

- Ask them to come up with three possible solutions that they think would be great for solving the problem.
- Ask your child to think deeply about each of the options for a minute and then analyze whether it is a great solution or not.
- After they are done with analyzing, ask him/her to select one from the solutions that they think would be perfect.
- Ask your child to try out the option to make sure it is going to solve the problem or not.

You will have to teach your child to start solving their own problems as this is the way they will be able to grow up in life and succeed. It can be regarded as a life process. It will never happen overnight, and so you will have to be patient with him/her. Also, you will have to instill self-reliance values so that your child can depend on themselves for solving all sorts of problems. In case you think your child is showcasing some kind of behavior that is out of control, do not opt for punishing him/her. You will also have to make your child understand that once they get self-reliant, it does not indicate that they cannot ask for other's help. Whenever they feel stuck somewhere, he/she can always ask out for help from all those who they trust.

If your child is facing difficulties in determining solutions by thinking, you can ask him/her to start writing down the solutions. It can act as a brainstorming session. If he/she has a bad mood, you will have to make them understand the importance of staying positive. Teach them how to say positive things, which can help in controlling their mood. In this way, they will get used to self-control when you are not present there to help them out. In simple terms, make them understand how they can give a positive pep talk to themselves. Dealing with all such problems, along with instilling good behavior, is more or less like developing new habits. So, the process of habit formation is not going to be easy. You will have to maintain consistency to make the whole process a grand success for the betterment of your child.

Chapter 6: Practical Tips for Dealing With Problems in School

Every child faces some sort of problems or the other during their school days. However, the problems of children who are suffering from the symptoms of ADHD are completely different from that of others. It is because the primary problem related to ADHD is that the affected children cannot properly concentrate or just maintain their focus on one thing for a long time. When you are in school, you have to maintain focus and be attentive as much as you can. Your children are expected to abide by the school rules. The teachers expect them to stay tidy and neat while maintaining a good connection with other children. We will discuss some of the widely found problems faced by ADHD children in school in this chapter and how they can be easily dealt with by both teachers and parents.

Enhancing Social Skills

The aspect of social skills is required to be stressed upon after your child starts attending school. Children suffering from the symptoms of ADHD tend to face problems as they are not easily accepted in their peer groups easily. Also, they do not come with the ability to make companions. They cannot show positivity as they connect with other people or children in school as they possess inattentive and hyperactive attitude. However, there are certain simple things that can be done on your part as parents to enhance the social skills of your child.

Teaching the Required Skills and Practicing

Regardless of the number of past experiences that your child has, you will notice that when he/she is suffering from the symptoms of ADHD, they are unable to learn from their past mistakes. They do not even think about the related consequences before they react. That is the reason why, every time when they showcase any kind of unacceptable behavior, you will have to take your stand and provide them with feedback. Make them know that their actions or behavior was not right for that very situation. One of the great ways of doing so is by engaging in activities of role-playing in social settings. It can be regarded as the best way to teach appropriate social skills to an ADHD child. You can also opt for teaching them how to react to bullies or teasing in school, which might otherwise result in being a hard situation for your child to handle.

Never try to do many things at one time. Try to start with only some areas of the problem so that it does not make your child feel overwhelmed during the process. For instance, children suffering from ADHD tend to face problems in initiating conversations or even properly maintain one. So, you can opt for teaching them how to maintain reciprocity in conversations. Next, you can move on to the ways in which they can resolve any kind of conflict in school in case they arise. You will also have to teach your child to develop healthy boundaries in some situations so that they can protect their personal space. Even children suffering from ADHD find it tough to speak in their normal voice. So, it is your responsibility to make your child understand what a normal tone is and what is said to be too loud. After you are done teaching all these skills to your child, you will have to make them practice all these skills over and over again so that it turns out to be a natural thing for them.

Enhancing Social Awareness

It has been found that ADHD children cannot really keep track of their social behaviors. In simple terms, they cannot be considered aware socially. They do not have any proper idea regarding how bad they can make other people feel with all their wrong actions. Also, they do not have any kind of understanding regarding their behavior that they should showcase in social settings. In some cases, when they interact with a peer, they might feel that everything went great. However, in actuality, it was far away from being considered as 'good.' So, it can be said that ADHD children have problems when it is all about reading situations properly. Thus, they end up assessing everything in the wrong way. This, in turn, results in incorrect self-evaluation. You will have to make your ADHD child understand all of these necessary skills.

Working on Development of Friendship

Everyone in this world needs friends, and so the same thing applies to your ADHD child too. However, they tend to face some serious problems when it comes to the aspect of making new friends. One of the amazing ways to ensure that he/she makes some nice friends is by sending them on playdates. It will also let you teach your child positive peer skills. Going on play dates will provide your child with the perfect chance to put all their positive peer skills to test. However, it will be better for you if you do not send your child for group activities from the very beginning. You can set a routine of playtime for your child with two to three other children. You will also have to keep in mind that the playdate length plays a significant role here. Children suffering from ADHD cannot get along well on long play dates.

In case your child is struggling with interactions in social settings, the period of middle and high school will tend to be very hard for them. That is why you will need to ensure that your child has a minimum of one good friend. It is because when your child does not have friends at all, social isolation of this nature might fuel them into developing friendships with all those children who might have some sort of negative influence on your child. It is quite a common thing in middle school and high school. You might even encourage your ADHD child to be a member of groups or communities where they can get the chance to nurture positive peer relationships. But the group in which you will enlist your child, you will need to ensure that the leader of the group is totally aware of the ADHD symptoms of your child. Also, it is of prime importance for the group leader to know how to deal with ADHD children.

Working With School for Making the Status of Peer Better

Problems might turn out to be worse for a child who is suffering from ADHD once they get labeled in some improper way by their peer group at school. Their reputation tends to remain the same for the majority of their life which might make it tough for them to go through their daily life. It will be a tough job to encourage your child in the direction of social relationships once he/she gets some kind of negative reputation for anything. To deal with such reputational effects, it will be better for you if you can reach out to your child's school and work in collaboration with the coaches or teachers. It is necessary to maintain a positive relationship with your child's teacher. You will also need to inform them regarding your child's ADHD along with the strengths and interests of your child. You will need to inform them of the main pain points of your child. Also, if you know some sort of strategy that worked really well for your child, make sure to let the teacher know everything about the same.

When your ADHD child is in kindergarten, it is quite natural for them to look out for their teacher when they are unable to figure out something or figure out whom they can be friends with. If the teacher can redirect your child in a proper and gentle way, along with warmth and acceptance, your child will be able to make friends easily. The social status of your child can be lifted up with the help of the teacher at least. The teachers of your child can also find someone in the class who is compassionate and pair up your child with the same person in order to make sure that your child can get social acceptance. To properly improve the classroom environment and also to make it friendly for your child, you will have to work in collaboration with your child's teacher.

How Can Teachers Help in Enhancing Social Competencies?

Your child gets in touch with the teacher on a daily basis in their school. It is the teacher who serves the responsibility of regulating the student's behavior in class. So, there are some specific things that can be done on the part of the teacher to enhance social competencies.

- The teacher can teach them the correct skills to improve the social awareness of the student. They will have to provide the students with positive attention and also show them the meaning of pro-social behavior. All of this requires to be done not only within the boundary of the classroom but also outside the boundary of the classroom.

- Whenever the child makes some mistake or does something wrong, it is the duty of the teacher to correct them by helping them with proper feedback. But one thing that the teacher will have to keep in mind is that the feedback provided by him/her should not be judgmental or embarrassing. The main aim of the teacher should be to build positive social skills for the concerned child.
- Whenever teachers come to find that one child is quite weak on the part of social skills, they can pair that child in supportive groups where no one will be teasing the child. Children who tend to be isolated socially need help in terms of friendships. The teacher will have to find friendships for the child.
- When children get engaged in cooperative behavior, the teacher can take their photos and just hang them in such places that can be seen easily in the classroom. It can help in encouraging positivity.

Rules and Expectations Needs to Be Realistic

If you want your ADHD child to be attentive and do well in school and also meet success, you will have to make sure that the rules and expectations that you set for them are realistic. The developmental delay in ADHD children is a huge factor that needs to be considered when both teachers and parents are setting up rules for them. The challenges faced by the child need to be accommodated, and that is the way all the rules should be set up. The primary difficulties that are faced by ADHD children that you need to keep in mind while setting up expectations and rules are:

- Problems in remembering routines or following directions or steps that they are asked to abide
- Recalling any kind of instruction that they were provided with to finish a task
- Time management
- Understanding what they should do with observation alone
- Emotion regulation
- Distractions and after they get distracted, properly figuring out their way back to the starting point of the discussion
- Navigating all the problems that come in their way

However, there are certain ways in which you can maintain your rules and expectations within the predictable and realistic boundary for your ADHD child.

- Usage of simple language and implementation of techqniues of hands-on teaching
- To make your child succeed despite all the challenges faced by him/her, you can opt for time manipulation at times. Also, you can opt to avoid any kind of hectic job for your ADHD child right away as they wake up in the morning. It will make sure that their energy does not get drained right at the beginning of the day. You might also wait until the ADHD medications start showing any kind of effect on your ADHD child before you can urge them to follow a routine.
- To make all kinds of tasks easier for the child, try to provide them with worksheets that can provide them with visual support and also provide them with all the steps that they need to follow. They will get the chance to achieve complex goals easily. Also, it will be on your part to order all the related steps properly so that your child does not get lost while figuring out which task to opt for first.

- In case you do not want your child to be on time, you can provide him/her with some sort of visual timer.
- Whenever your child starts getting lost on their way, you can provide them with gentle prompts or redirections.
- You can develop an incentive program so that it can help in the promotion of good behavior on the part of your child.
- Positive expectations and enforcements will have to be of consistent nature.
- If your child is sad or anxious, try to listen to what they have to say and just empathize with him/her. They will start feeling understood in this way, and all their emotions will slowly calm down.
- If nothing goes according to the plan, you will have to acknowledge the same in front of your ADHD child that it is completely okay at times if things fail to turn out the way they should. It is because there are various circumstances that are at play, and your child might just override the expectations and rules.
- In case you have decided to reward your child for showing good behavior, try to make it consistent as well; otherwise, your child might just not understand what your expectations are and will start getting mixed messages.

Managing Distractibility

Distraction is a thing that is common among every ADHD child. It is something that every ADHD child has to fight with. When children suffering from ADHD are at school, it is the responsibility of the teachers to handle their distractions. It is mainly because, when they get distracted, they will not be taking any information that is being shared in the classroom as their mind will be present somewhere else. In case the task at hand needs excessive mental effort, the distractions might turn out to be stronger. Sometimes you might feel that your child is properly listening to you. However, in actuality, nothing is going through their ears. All that they are trying to do is to pretend that they are listening to you. But they just cannot retain any information. Anything like someone passing through the hallway beside their classroom or chirping birds in the trees nearby can easily distract an ADHD child.

There are certain very easy things that can be done on your part. The first thing is not to allow them to opt for a long time of work. In place of that, you can just break down all those periods into several small chunks. There are some other strategies as well that can help in the betterment of your ADHD child.

- Ensure that your child is not seated at a place where there are doors and windows nearby. In case you want your

child to be focused at home, you will have to ensure that there are no pets in the room as your child is trying to pay attention to something.
- Every kind of important and necessary information needs to be provided to the ADHD child in written format. You can also opt for a checklist or to-do-list for your child where he/she can notice without any effort, such as a bulletin board in class. You will also have to remind your child that the teacher will put up important information on the board from time to time.
- Discuss with the teacher and ask them not to conduct seated activities for a long time for your child. The teacher can easily alter the times with all those activities that need your child to show some sort of physical movement or move around in the room.
- In case there is any big assignment that needs to be completed, try to divide the same into multiple small chunks. Ask the teacher to give some break to your child when they are done with one chunk of task.

Management of Impulsivity

Whenever any nature of difficult social situation tends to arise, you will see that ADH children start acting out. Also, they might not just think before doing or saying anything. It is what is known as trouble with impulse control. It is also the reason why ADHD children are most often tagged as rube or unruly. The problem of impulsivity might result in a series of problems for the child when he/she is at school. However, you can opt for imposing certain behavior plans to make them feel that they have total control of the day. It will help in avoiding the feeling of insecurity that is often considered as the main cause of impulsivity. There are certain essential things that can be done on your part.

- As already said before, things that are written tend to have more impact on ADHD children in comparison to verbal instructions. So, you can write down some particular behavioral plan for the child and ask his/her teacher to attach the same to their desk.
- When the child showcases good behavior, try not to praise them privately. Try to praise him/her out loud right in front of others. It will provide them with the idea of what is right and what is wrong.
- When you notice some sort of misbehavior from the child, try to state to them the consequences of the same clearly. To properly make your child realize that what has been done on their part is considered misbehavior, you will

need to be as detailed as possible as you state the related consequences.
- Try to write down the whole day schedule of your child. Whenever he/she gets done with something, just cross off that particular item from the schedule. It will help in imparting a sense of control on the kid, which might also help in making the child calmer.

Reduction of Interruptions

Like we have discussed multiple times before, children who suffer from the symptoms of ADHD tend to face lots of problems with controlling their impulses. So, at the time of teaching, the child might start speaking out of turn when the teacher is teaching something. It can be noticed at home as well when the child starts speaking when they are not meant to. At times, whatever is being said by the child might not just be considered to be normal and might somewhat be equal to an outburst. In some cases, in fact, such outbursts might turn out to be aggressive and rude. All of this might result in the creation of a wide range of problems for the child when they are in the classroom. It might not even allow them to socialize with other children. Additionally, children suffering from ADHD come with very low self-esteem that tends to make everything even worse for them.

In case the teacher tries to point out that the child is behaving in a wrong way or they are undisciplined right in front of the whole class, the child might just take it to hurt. In such a case, the situation might just go out of control. That is the reason why you will have to develop a nature of talk that can be understood only by the child and you. It can be treated as a 'secret language.' You can ask the teachers of your child to adopt the same. As long as the teachers can properly communicate with the child that are creating interruptions, however, in a discreet manner, everything should be fine. On the other hand, when the teacher can take a class without any form of interruption from the part of the ADHD child, the teacher should praise him/her.

Management of Hyperactivity

You must have noticed that when a child is suffering from the symptoms of ADHD, they will have the tendency to be in motion constantly. They might keep on fighting with other children in the classroom, fidgeting, kick out things, or just show some sort of movement all the time. Well, there are various creative ways in which the teacher can help the child to properly manage their hyperactivity. When an ADHD child is taught to channelize their energy in various ways, they can be attentive and remain focused when they need to do some kind of work. Release of this form of energy is very important in case you want the child to calm down. There are some strategies that you can follow.

- The teacher can just send the child on an errand. Ask the teacher of your child to provide them with some sort of task that the child can complete for the teacher. It might be as simple as sharpening some pencils, or just bring about some books from the other class. The child might also be asked to distribute worksheets or workbooks in the classroom or just bring some chalks from the faculty room.
- A great way in which teachers can manage the hyperactivity of ADHD children is by making them engaged in some kind of sport. It can be as simple as running around the field. Also, it should be the teacher's duty to make sure that the child does not skip the class of physical education.
- As a parent, all that you can do is to limit the time that your child spends watching TV. Encourage him/her to go outside and get indulged in some sort of physical activity. It can help in preventing your child from being hyperactive in their school.
- Also, providing ADHD children with some sort of stress-relieving objects, such as a stress ball, can help a lot. It can be done when they are seated in the classroom. Pressing and squeezing the

stress ball can help in releasing their extra energy, by which their hyperactive symptoms can be suppressed.

Making the Task of Learning Fun

If you really want your child to be attentive towards their academics and to learn new things, you will have to pay attention to making the whole thing fun. You can start by providing him/her with some interesting trivia, or just opt for playing some funny videos which are educational in nature. You might also opt for singing silly songs so that your child can easily remember all those stuff from the boring subjects. Concepts of mathematics are one of the toughest things that can be inculcated in an ADHD child. That is the reason why using games for making the whole process a fun thing is a great option. There are some other ideas as well that you can opt for.

- There is a wide range of games that you can play with your child. To make the concept of numbers a bit fun, you can opt for dice, dominoes, or memory cards. In case you do not have any of these, there is nothing to worry about as there are several ways in which you will not need to have anything. For instance, you can use your fingers and toes and just tuck them in as you are adding or subtracting.

- In case you are solving word problems with your child, you can opt for drawing some pictures to make the entire process a lot more interesting. Concepts of mathematics can be easily understood if you try to illustrate everything to your ADHD child. For instance, if the problem says that you have ten apples, you can draw ten apples on the notebook and also encourage your child to do the same.
- If there is a big phrase or word that your ADHD child has to keep in mind, you can opt for some acronyms for the same that are funny. They will be able to remember the words easily with this technique.

The next big thing that you will have to teach your child is to read properly. For ADHD children, reading properly might also turn out to be a tough task as they find it difficult to stay focused on one thing for a prolonged time. You can start by providing him/her with some interesting storybooks or factual books, something in which they can find interest. Here are certain things that can be done to make the whole process a lot easier:

- You can read out stories to your child as a parent. It will also permit you to have some quality time with him/her.
- You can opt for acting out the story to make the whole thing interesting and

funny. Try to use funny voices and make some costumes.
- As you read out a story to your child, you can ask him/her what they think will happen next in the story.

Try to encourage your child to get done with their homework in the correct way. However, for that, you will also have to make your child organized by opting for color-coding the subjects. It will help in ensuring that your child does not get overwhelmed with the provided amount of homework that they have to finish. Try not to make your child do the homework for a long time continuously. For instance, if he/she is doing their homework for half an hour, try to give them a short break for ten minutes. Also, breaks that include sipping water or their favorite milkshake or going to the washroom or favorite milkshake can also help in boosting the whole process of studying.

Chapter 7: Managing ADHD Behavior Outside the Boundary of School

Your child cannot be at home all the time, and there are various other places where he/she will have to go apart from their school. It is your responsibility to teach your ADHD child to properly manage all their behavior in every other place as well. Well, this chapter will be helpful for all those parents who are planning to go on a family trip with their ADHD child.

Traveling By Car

One of the primary things that most ADHD children dread is traveling by car. It might turn out to be a challenge for the parents as well. It is because children who are the victims of the symptoms of ADHD generally prefer to be in their routines only. Their sense of order might get easily hampered by simple out-of-the routine things, such as long rides by car. All of this can result in a phase of tantrums and turmoil. The ultimate result of this is that the family finds it tough to travel anywhere by car anymore. However, in this section, you will come across some simple suggestions that might help you in making your experience of traveling by car with your ADHD child a better one the next time.

- In case you are going somewhere with your child that involves traveling by car, you will have to prepare him/her mentally before few days of going for the trip. You just cannot wake up one morning and tell your child that you will be traveling somewhere that will involve traveling by car for four to five hours or even more than that. You will need to prepare your ADHD child for the alteration of routine along with the scenery that is going to come. If you really want your child to make him/her feel at home even while traveling, you will have to accept all their suggestions regarding all those things that they would like to carry with them. You will also have to explain to your child the motive of the trip or the destination that you have decided to travel to. Also, you can tell him/her about the road and the sceneries that they can enjoy at the time of travel. In this way, you will get the chance to prepare your child mentally for the trip.

- Try to maintain at least some portions of their daily routine as you travel. For instance, try to wake up your child at the same time as they do every day. If you just try to wake up your child one hour before one or two hours of their daily time, he/she might not be in a good mood. In fact, the chances of them throwing tantrums might also be high. So, try to avoid scheduling all your trips that are way ahead of the daily routine of your child.

- In case the overall time of traveling by car is quite long, your ADHD child might like to take a short nap. However, they are used to sleeping in their bed, and sleeping in the car might seem odd to them. So, it would be a superb idea if you can bring their favorite blanket or favorite stuffed toy in order to make them feel comfortable in the car. ADHD children tend to feel secure by the sense of familiarity.

- If he/she starts looking exhausted or tired after a certain point of time, opt for taking a break and just stop somewhere. When your child fails to have enough sleep, the ADHD symptoms might start worsening. You cannot just let that happen, specifically when you are traveling. So, try to encourage your child to take small naps if you are traveling for a long time or in case you still have some great amount of distance to cover.

- Try not to change the determined behavioral rules. You will have to make him/her realize that only because they are not at home and traveling somewhere by car does not provide them a free pass to do anything they feel like. In case he/she starts misbehaving, ensure that you remind them of the related consequences.

- There are several simple things that actually matter when you have decided to travel with your ADHD child by car. He/she might just not comply with all that you say or as simple as putting on the seatbelt. In case your child is not at all listening to you, try not to jump to the system of getting them reminded of the consequences right away. In place of doing that, understand why he/she is actually acting grumpy. In order to keep your ADHD child cheerful, you can try to make them a part of the conversation that you are having with other family members.

- You will also need to maintain the social etiquette of your child whenever you are traveling outside. You can opt for giving your child gentle reminders and just follow the process of reminding them of the related consequences in case they keep behaving rudely.

- A very common commotion that ADHD children have at the time of traveling by car is the seating arrangement.

Sometimes, children might have some special preferences for their seating. They might even get moody in case they are not permitted to sit in their preferred seat. You will need to teach them how they can share and also maintain a mutual seating arrangement.

- Another common problem that tends to arise on road trips with ADHD children is the part of going to the washroom. In case the trip is long, it is quite a natural thing for you to stop for washroom breaks. At first, your child might want to go to the washroom as you want to go. However, soon after that, they might start throwing tantrums regarding going to the washroom right away. That is the reason why you will have to ensure that your child gets done with their washroom activities right before you leave so that there is no need for them to go to the washroom anytime soon. Even if he/she wants to go to the washroom after some time, make them know that it is tough to locate a toilet on the road. So, they will need to wait for some time depending on the availability of washrooms and the road.

How to Deal With Your Child's Bad Behavior in Public Settings?

Do you always feel tensed and worried regarding the tantrums that you think your ADHD child might throw whenever you go to a public place with him/her? Behavior turns out to be a serious issue with children suffering from the symptoms of ADHD. No matter whatever you ask them to do that they actually do not want to, he/she might just lash out in an aggressive way at you. Whenever an ADHD child is overpowered with an array of strong emotions that they might not deal with until and unless they showcase some form of emotional outburst or act out. However, you will have to do something regarding their misbehavior right now as otherwise, in case it gets neglected and gets fostered, after a period of time, your ADHD child might just develop an oppositional defiant disorder or ODD. Also, according to some reports, ODD has been found in about 40% of children who are suffering from the symptoms of ADHD.

Why Does ADHD Children Act Out?

Right before we delve deeper into the management of behavioral patterns of ADHD children, you will have to understand why do they act out in the first place. Try to think about the history of ADHD of your child and the ways in which they have been fighting to deal with the same since childhood. In fact, it has been found that children suffering from

ADHD tend to get attracted to all those things which they should just stay away from. For instance, if you ask your child to behave properly, he/she might just get attracted to all forms of malicious intent. That is the main reason why, whenever you are out in public with your ADHD child, and you ask him/her to sit in one place, they would just run around that place or start speaking loudly. All of this can easily make you feel stressed in public settings. In fact, it is because of all such situations that result in negative interactions between the ADHD child and you.

As you keep telling your child from an early stage during their childhood that behavior of this sort is not right and they should stay from them, the child might just start feeling that there must be something wrong with them. So, they just start internalizing all the feelings that they have. At times, they might just act out towards all those people who ask them to stay away from such behaviors or things.

Reasons Why ADHD Children Throw Tantrums

In the last section, we have discussed in detail the reasons why ADHD children tend to act out. Now, we will discuss the reasons why they opt for throwing tantrums. Children suffering from the symptoms of ADHD usually have to give in a lot of extra effort in getting things done that seem repetitive or boring to them. It indicates that he/she has to deal with a lot of resistance, which makes all their tasks more challenging automatically. In case the task is not permitting them to opt for things that they love or like, for instance, watching TV, they might just decide not to do the task at all. This, in turn, would take the shape of a battleground. These are nothing but strategies of avoidance that your ADHD child tries to opt for. However, for you, they just turn into power struggles quickly, along with being acts of defiance.

When your ADHD child starts throwing tantrums, you might make up your mind to alter the conditions of the overall task so that all of it gets easier for him/her. All of this will make your child feel that they have got the power to throw unnecessary tantrums any time they feel like as you keep reducing conditions for the sake of them.

Strategies to Deal With Tantrums

Let us now discuss the various ways in which you can keep the bad behaviors of your ADHD child under proper control. All forms of disciplinary strategies that are used for other kids might just not work for children who are suffering from the symptoms of ADHD. It is because of one primary reason – you have already developed some form of negative interaction with your child. In fact, if you truly want the strategies to function in the best way for your child, you will have to keep your temper under control. If your ADHD child does not showcase bad behavior every now and then, then raising your voice or just speaking to them firmly might work for bringing them back on track. However, the main problem lies with all those ADHD children who have imbibed it as a habit to misbehave. If you just keep raising your voice or shout at them as you talk, they just think of that to be normal. So, they will just stop paying any form of attention to whatever you do.

Additionally, when you opt for giving too much punishment, the effectiveness of all of that will soon disappear. They will assume that they are living in a world of perpetual punishment, and so it will slowly lose all its meaning. He/she might not just think of it as a big deal when you punish them, and so there will be no effect if they get punished one more time. However, in order to bring your child on track, something can be done on your part.

- When you succeed in introducing a structured routine or lifestyle in the life of your ADHD child, it has been found that he/she might get some sort of benefit from the same. It indicates that you will have to provide them with a proper set of directions or instructions whenever you want your child to do something. You will have to aim towards writing down everything that you are actually expecting from your ADHD child so that they get aware of the same. In case you fail to make your child understand which behaviors are correct and which behaviors are not, how are they going to differentiate between right and wrong?

- There is a very common term that all of you must have heard – scaffolding. In case a child is facing some sort of behavioral problems, then to properly regulate their behavior, they will need a perfect family environment. Also, if you want your ADHD child to learn something great in life, you will have to provide him/her with a proper structure to do so.

- You will need to develop a positive relationship with your ADHD child. The importance of this tends to increase if you want to mend the disruptive behavior of him/her. It is because when there is a bad relationship between the parent and the child, everything seems to be negative. And thus, the disruptive behaviors will just tend to escalate.

- One of the primary reasons why ADHD children showcase bad behaviors is that they are unable to regulate their emotions. So, you will have to work with your child in order to make them more aware of all their emotions. You will also need to teach them the ways in which they can practice self-control. We have already discussed self-control in Chapter 5.

Helping Your ADHD Child in Group Situations

There will be a number of situations where your ADHD child will need to work in collaboration in a group. It might be in their school or even at some party or when they decide to go out and play with other children. However, navigating in this sort of group situation is something that the majority of ADHD children face a problem with. Also, if a proper form of care is not taken, the situation might escalate quite quickly. In the end, the overall group exercise will just leave a negative nature of impact on your ADHD child. Similar to other children, if someone is suffering from the symptoms of ADHD, it does not hamper their desire to make new friends, or be a part of group activities, or even succeed in life. In order to help your child with the same, there are certain things that you will have to do to help him/her.

- Indeed, most of the parents are well aware of the fact that ADHD is a true disorder, and they will have to deal with the same with proper care. However, there are still groups of parents who do not tend to believe in the existence of this disorder. You will have to understand that the symptoms of ADHD in your child are not at all a result of your upbringing. It is nothing more than a disorder in the brain, and it also does not reflect the intelligence of your child. When you try to think that the symptoms of ADHD are not serious at all, you might just start taking all their bad behaviors and tantrums as being willful. All of this can easily make the situation worse.

- You will need to develop a routine before changing the gears. In case you have decided to take things to a higher level in group activities, provide your ADHD child with proper time to prepare for the same.

- To properly deal with all the extra energy that is possessed by your ADHD child, it is your duty to encourage them in various forms of positive opportunities in which they can spend all their energy. As you try to channelize the energy of your ADHD child towards something positive, the chances of them misbehaving or acting out will be less.

- There are some correction strategies that you will have to use as they will help your ADHD child with all their group activities. Try not to criticize anything that he/she does. When your child finally starts taking their steps in the correct direction, you will have to appreciate them in place of just telling them the ways how they can be more perfect. There is no need to push your child in the direction of perfectionism as they are not required to be perfect. All that they need to do is to just continue with all that they are doing.

- At times, you will find that your child is acting out aggressively. However, they do not mean most of the things that they say. It is because their self-control level is low. However, it does not indicate that they will be willing to emotionally hurt you. So, ensure that your reaction to anything is calm. Try not to act out immediately to make them understand by using some form of punishment.

- Try not to be attentive to the negatives. For instance, do not keep telling them all the time what they are not supposed to do. It is because your child might start feeling restrictive. Try to tell them all those things that they should actually do. It will help in the promotion of positive activity in him/her.

- If your ADHD child has been harnessing negative energy, you can just ask him/her to get some simple chores done for you so that all forms of negative energy get out of their body and mind.

- Try to refrain from accusing your ADHD child of anything. You will need to understand and accept the very fact that your child is a slow learner. You will have to provide them with all the time he/she needs. There is no use in pushing them towards something within a fixed timeframe. They will take the time they need, no matter what.

It is a true fact that going outside with your child who is suffering from the symptoms of ADHD is a challenging task. It is mainly because their mood will keep changing all the time during the course of the day. He/she might be excessively happy now and just get sad in the next moment. Also, children suffering from ADHD come with a low level of tolerance. So, they are most likely to get frustrated easily. However, if you start following the steps that we have discussed in this chapter, you can easily learn to navigate slowly through all types of situations.

Chapter 8: Using Medication for Treating ADHD

There is a very common question that comes in the minds of most parents – "Is it okay to opt for medications to treat ADHD?" or "Do all these medications come with any kind of side effects?" It is quite natural to have all these questions in your mind when you have to deal with the tantrums of your child, being an ADHD child-parent. We will address all these questions in detail in this chapter. Indeed, the related symptoms of ADHD can be easily kept under control by the use of medications. It applies both to children and adults. You can easily get a hold of the inattentiveness, impulsivity, and hyperactivity of your ADHD child by opting for the right medications. However, there are certain things that you will have to keep in mind. First, medication is not a permanent solution for ADHD. Second, you will have to understand that are a number of side effects and risks that come along with all these medications.

In fact, if you have gone through the first chapter of this book, you already know that medication is not the one and only form of treating ADHD. No matter if you are the victim of ADHD itself or it is about your child, it is essential to get all knowledge regarding ADHD medications. Getting comprehensive knowledge will make sure that you opt for the right decisions and also go for the best options. Before we jump right into the details, we will have to first understand how medications can help a child suffering from ADHD and also what their limitations are. Taking the correct medications will help the patient to stay focused on all the tasks that they have in hand, get control over their impulses, and also plan everything properly. However, you will also need to keep in mind that medications won't work like magic. You might see that your child is still suffering from various symptoms like forgetfulness and social anxiety from time to time, even after having the medications.

So, several other changes in the regular lifestyle of your ADHD child are needed for imparting any form of long-term change. It also includes maintaining a good sleep cycle, opting for daily exercise, and a healthy diet as well. Always remember that regardless of the type of medication prescribed to your child, ADHD will be a lifelong problem. It cannot be cured with the help of medications. However, when medications are administered, you can easily get some relief from the repeating symptoms of your child. There are parents who think that as now their children are not showcasing any kind of symptoms, the time has come to stop the medications. However, the moment it is done, the symptoms just come back, and even in worse conditions. Also, you will have to keep in mind that the medications might not just work in the same way for every child. If someone else's child is benefitting from a certain medicine, it does not indicate that it will work the same for your child as well.

The reaction of an ADHD child to a particular medicine is actually unpredictable. It is because every human being shows different responses to different medications. That is the reason why when you will take your ADHD child to a doctor; they will diagnose him/her, determine the type and intensity of the symptoms of your child, and then administer a dosage that is only meant for your child. In simple terms, the medications prescribed for ADHD are very much personalized. Also, you will have to take your child for regular checkups so that the symptoms do not go out of hand.

Stimulant Medicines

There are two groups of medications that are widely used in treating ADHD in children. One of them is stimulant medicines. Such medications generally help in dealing with hyperactivity, stretching your child's span of short attention, and controlling impulsive behavior. At times, doctors might just opt for treating patients solely based on stimulant medications. At other times, therapy might also be prescribed along with medication. It has been found that approximately 80% of the children tend to see improvement in their symptoms with the usage of stimulant medications. In fact, such medicines can also help in improving your relationship with your child. If your child keeps taking the medicines without any fail, then you will notice not only great behavioral tendencies but also more attention on their part. But there is still a lack of evidence to prove that stimulant medications can help in controlling the social life of ADHD children.

One more fact that you will have to keep in mind regarding stimulant medicines is that they are being used for the treatment of ADHD for the longest time. The overall effectiveness of such medicines in treating ADHD children is also backed up by a number of studies. Some of the common names in this group of medicine include Adderall, Ritalin, and Dexedrine.

Non-Stimulant Medicines

In the last section, we discussed stimulant medications. However, they are not the only kind of drug that can be used for controlling the symptoms of ADHD. One more kind of drug is also used and is known as non-stimulant medication. It includes a wide range of medicines that are used as antidepressants, for controlling blood pressure, and even Strattera. Generally, doctors try not to prescribe non-stimulant medicines right away. The very first choice that is opted by most doctors is stimulant medication. However, if stimulant medicines cannot be prescribed to some children because of some pre-existing health-related problems or if the stimulant medication fails to show any kind of result, then only non-stimulant medications are prescribed by doctors. Let us discuss the non-stimulant medicines one by one.

Strattera: It is a commonly used non-stimulant medicine that is prescribed by doctors. In fact, this medicine has been approved by the FDA. The medicine is popularly known by the generic name – atomoxetine. The levels of dopamine in the brain get affected by stimulant medications. However, in the case of this medicine, it affects the levels of norepinephrine by increasing the same. In comparison to other types of non-stimulant medicines, it has been found that the overall effect of Strattera tends to be more than others. Additionally, you will be able to get relief from the symptoms of your ADHD child for one whole day. So, for all those ADHD children who face difficulties in waking up in the morning, this medicine is a superb option. Another plus point regarding Strattera is that it can help in dealing with depression.

In case your ADHD child is also dealing with depression, this medication can be regarded as a good option for him/her. Besides all of this, the overall effectiveness of Strattera for treating ADHD symptoms in children is much better than other medications. However, there might be some common side effects, such as nausea, vomiting, mood swings, upset stomach, abdominal pain, headache, dizziness, and sleepiness. Now let us have a look at another type of non-stimulant medication that is used for treating the symptoms of ADHD. However, this medication is not FDA approved and is generally 'off-label.'

Antidepressants: It is prescribed for all those patients with ADHD who are also dealing with depression. The types of antidepressants that are generally administered in these cases tend to target more than one neurotransmitter. A very common antidepressant is Wellbutrin. The generic name of this medication is Bupropion. The aim of this medicine is both norepinephrine and dopamine. Besides this, there is one more line of treatment that is open for the doctors, which generally involves the usage of tricyclic antidepressants. The related side effects are quite mild. However, the patient might start experiencing irritability, loss of appetite, and decreased sleep.

Medicines for high blood pressure:
Besides the first two options, this medicine is also prescribed for treating ADHD. However, not every medication of this category can be regarded as suitable for the treatment of ADHD. Some of the common medicines include Tenex and Catapres.

Chapter 9: Suggestions and Tips for Parenting ADHD Child

In this book, we have discussed the various types of problems and challenges that might be faced by your ADHD child, and we have also discussed various solutions for the same. The overall process might seem quite overwhelming and might even turn out to be frustrating at times. However, as you are the parent, you will have to take up the responsibility of teaching your ADHD child how they can properly navigate through all these issues. You will have to make him/her understand how all such problems can be overcome. The earlier you can recognize all such problems and also address them, the chances of your child being happier in their later life will also increase.

Making It Interesting

Distraction is one of the primary problems that are faced by almost every child suffering from the symptoms of ADHD. Even the minute things can distract them from their tasks. However, in some cases, the ADHD child might get way too focused on any task that you provide them. It is known as being hyper-focused. In case you want your ADHD child to not get distracted and also retain their focus on the task that they have in hand, make sure that the task is not boring. Even if the texts in their books are boring, it will be your duty to use drawings or some other forms of visuals so that it can be made interesting for your child.

Teaching Time Management

Children suffering from the symptoms of ADHD tend to take forever to complete even the simplest work in their daily lives. It is something that you will have to work on to improve as a parent. In case you just try to him/her do the tasks forcefully while thinking that it is the only solution, you will be doing it wrong. It is because as you try to enforce something on your child, it will only be aggravating the overall problem. Once you can teach your ADHD child how to properly manage their time, everything will be just more manageable. In fact, they will be able to navigate through all their issues with ease.

- Well, I cannot really stress enough the importance of daily routine for your ADHD child. Indeed, a proper routine can help in solving a wide range of problems in their lives. You will need to think about the primary responsibilities that your child has first and then start making the routine. However, you will have to keep in mind that the routine cannot be made entirely of tasks that you want your child to get done with.

You will have to leave enough time for other activities, along with sufficient breaks. Also, you will have to maintain some sameness as you schedule their routine. For example, if you have scheduled your child's playtime at 04:30 PM on Monday, ensure that it is the same on Tuesday as well. It will help in giving some structure to the life of your ADHD child.

- You will need to work on discarding any form of dawdling. Make sure you keep checking your child to stay away from such incidences. You will need to stick to all those times that you have scheduled for each of their activities. In fact, you can also start using a timer for proper enforcement of all those times. In order to encourage positive behavior, you can also opt for an incentive-based program.

Reminding Yourself That It Is Not Only Your Child Who Misbehaves

With all sorts of challenges that tend to come in your way as you handle your child who is suffering from the symptoms of ADHD, you might just get lost in the flow quite easily. You will have to understand and also remind yourself that ADHD is not the root cause for all types of incorrect behaviors. If you believe that everything that is done by your child is the result of ADHD, then you might just let him/her get away with several things as they have ADHD. That is the reason why it is so important to make yourself clear that every child misbehaves at times, and there is no need to manage everything. Yes, it is true that certain types of behaviors are hard to be neglected. However, at the end of the day, you will have to figure out which behaviors need to be managed and which ones you can deal with some other day.

Approaching a Specialist for Getting Support

In case you are facing lots of difficulties, along with stress, while dealing with your ADHD child, then you might just need to take the help of a specialist. There are various support groups that you can opt for besides professional help. However, opting for the specialist will always seem like a huge task. The specialist that you will choose for your ADHD child needs to be someone with whom he/she can be comfortable. You can initiate the process by taking some recommendations from the general doctor of your child and then opt for an appointment with a specialist to find out whether your ADHD child likes him/her or not. Right before you can determine the correct fit, you might just need to visit a lot of them. Well, that is absolutely fine. Try not to settle for anything that you get as if you opt for the wrong specialist, your child might find it difficult to open to him/her. It will not be possible to develop a true relationship.

Being Calm

As you deal with all sorts of chaos by yourself, the internal balance might just get affected badly. You might soon start not feeling well. That is the reason why it is always advised to all the parents to stay calm if you want to properly handle your ADHD child. When you keep your mind calm, your brain can start thinking clearly, and every sort of problem can be solved easily.

Conclusion

Thank you very much for making it through right to the end portion of the Parenting ADHD; let's hope it was full of information and was also able to deliver you with all needed the tools that you require to attain your goals, regardless of what they may be.

All the suggestions and solutions that have been provided in this book focus only on one thing, and that is to provide your child with the required help. It is all about how your child can opt for effective self-control and self-care in all types of situations, despite their symptoms of ADHD. It is essential for dealing with the present of your child and also to have a healthy and bright future. If you just keep following all the recommended suggestions properly, you will be able to develop a very special bond with your ADHD child, a kind of relationship where both of you will respect each other. Try not to take excessive stress. All that you need to do is to stay calm and just keep implementing everything that you have learned from this book. You will soon notice that everything is perfectly falling into place.

Children suffering from the symptoms of ADHD already need to experience a great deal of stress in their daily lives as they try their best to cope up with everything that keeps happening around them. However, if you just abide by the strategies provided in this book, you will get the opportunity to make all their daily struggle a lot easier. Children are bound to struggle with being organized, getting done with the simplest tasks, or even remember stuff. But can never leave hope. You will have to keep full faith in your child and just make him/her complete things one at a time. The related symptoms of ADHD are different for every child. Some children might wake up with a bad mood in the morning, while some might have mood swings during the evening. You will have to properly monitor all the symptoms of your child and just think about the ways in which you can make the toughest days of your child a bit easier.

Children suffering from the symptoms of ADHD often feel cluttered. It can result in the creation of a great deal of confusion in your child, which might also make them overwhelmed. So, you will have to stress on being organized. It is quite essential if you want your child to get done with their studies properly and also finish all their tasks timely. There are certain things that you can do to keep your child organized.

- Try to use pocket folders of various colors. For instance, in the red colored folder, you can arrange all the homework assignments of your child. You can make another folder for

arranging all the papers that have been returned by the teachers and are graded. If your child has to deal with a great number of subjects, you can create various folders for different subjects in order to make things easier for them.
- You can also use color-coding to separate all those tasks that your child has to complete.

Also, it will be your duty to keep the study desk of your child completely organized so that your ADHD child wants to study. You can make your child understand the importance of being organized and make them clear all the clutter on their study table. You can also keep a basket beside the study desk so that he/she can throw away all the stuff that they do not need. You will have to make sure the place where your child studies have a fresh vibe. Also, the location needs to be comfortable for your child. As your child organizes his/her room, you can spend some time with them and make the whole thing turn into a fun activity.

Parents of ADHD children seem to be very over-protective. While doing so, you might just start thinking of other people as your enemy. However, in actuality, it is not so. You might get the feeling that the member of your family or people surrounding your ADHD child are not providing him/her with enough care. But you will need to understand that every individual comes with their own way of caring. However, if you strongly feel that some individual is not providing enough care to your child, you can opt for getting indulged in a proper form of communication. There is no need to treat that person as your enemy. You can simply converse with them regarding your child, the strengths and weaknesses of him/her, along with their preferences.

When you are with your ADHD child, who seems to be very hyperactive the majority of the time and also keeps showcasing impulsive behavior, it might result in a power struggle. It turns out to be more difficult when you have to deal with the same every day. In that case, you will need to learn to pick up your battles. Just do not answer every tantrum that is thrown by your ADHD child. If you fail to do so, you might end up feeling frustrated, while your child will think that they can do whatever they want. So, you will have to learn the ways in which you can let go of small things so that you can successfully alleviate your level of stress. Also, children suffering from ADHD cannot do well with direct commands. So, do not command your child to do something. Try to explain to him/her what needs to be done.

It is essential to dwell on positivity as you handle your ADHD child. You will have to provide them with feedback. Indeed, it might just seem impossible at times for you to focus on positivity. So, as a parent, you will have to develop an outlet where you can easily express all your concerns and worries. Try to opt for online groups if you need help of any kind.

Lastly, if you found this guidebook beneficial in any way, a nice review on Amazon is always valued!

Printed in Great Britain
by Amazon